The Calcium Key

The Revolutionary Diet Discovery That Will Help You Lose Weight Faster

Michael Zemel, Ph.D.

Bill Gottlieb

WILEY

John Wiley & Sons, Inc.

Published by John Wiley & Sons, Inc., Hoboken, New Jersey
Published simultaneously in Canada

Design and production by Navta Associates, Inc.

Library of Congress Cataloging-in-Publication Data:

Zemel, Michael B.
   The calcium key : the revolutionary diet discovery that will help you lose weight faster / Michael Zemel and Bill Gottlieb.
      p. cm.
Includes bibliographical references and index.
ISBN 0-471-46368-X (Cloth)
1. Weight loss. 2. Calcium–Metabolism–Regulation–Popular works.
I. Gottlieb, William, 1953- II. Title.
   RM222.2.Z455 2004
   613.2't—dc22

                                                   2003017783

Printed in the United States of America

10 9 8 7 6 5 4 3 2 1

AUTHOR'S NOTE

Although *The Calcium Key* is a collaborative effort by Michael B. Zemel, Ph.D., and Bill Gottlieb, we have used the pronoun *I* for Dr. Zemel throughout, because the book is based on his scientific research and perspectives.

At their request, the identities of the people described in the case histories have been changed to protect confidentiality.

To my children, Abby and Rachel,
my fiancée, Sharon,
and my mother,
for their love, support, and tolerance,
and to the memory of my father,
who always enthusiastically supported my scientific
and academic interests
but kept telling me that I should write a practical book . . .
I wish he could read this one.

Michael

For moistest-eyed Denise,
from her smiling cheese
lover,

Bill

Contents

Acknowledgments

We would like to acknowledge:

Our agent, Chris Tomasino, for her invaluable assistance in shaping the proposal of *The Calcium Key,* for selling it, and for continuing to advocate the success of the book in every way possible.

Our editor, Tom Miller, executive editor of General Interest Books at Wiley, for immediately understanding the significance of Dr. Zemel's discoveries, and for all his enthusiastic work with and on behalf of *The Calcium Key.*

Tammi Hancock, R.D., for developing the delicious recipes and easy-to-follow meal plans of the Calcium Key Weight-Loss Plan.

Sarah Russell, R.D., study coordinator, for her informative perspectives on the day-to-day implementation of the Calcium Key Exchange System, and for the help of the other staff members in the Nutrition and Metabolic Research Clinic at the University of Tennessee: Joanna Richards, R.N., Lea Gebhardt, M.S., R.D., Anita Milstead, R.D., and Danielle Morgan, R.D.

Dixie Thompson, Ph.D., F.A.C.S.M., for so generously giving of her expertise and time for chapter 6 on exercise in *The Calcium Key.*

The many individuals who lost weight on the Calcium Key Weight-Loss Plan while participating in research at the University of Tennessee, for sharing the inspiring stories of their weight-loss success.

Michael:

This project really started in 1988 with the accidental observation that dairy-rich diets produce significant loss of body fat. Moving from that observation to clear molecular and physiological explanations and to clinical confirmation of these concepts has been a long journey made possible only by the cooperation and interest of many colleagues. If I can borrow from the "It takes a village to raise a child" concept, it takes many scientists and many laboratories to raise a mature, useful idea. Unfortunately, I know that in listing names I risk omitting someone, and for that unintentional error I apologize in advance.

Prior to the "aha" moment in which we realized that there may indeed be a logical explanation for dairy regulation of fat metabolism, we spent a number of years working on the key regulatory molecular and biochemical systems in fat cells that serve as the basis for our dietary findings. This work involved a number of key players to whom I am grateful. Dr. Richard Woychik and his colleagues initially cloned the *agouti* gene described in chapter 1, and it was through initial discussions and collaboration with Dr. Woychik that we developed a mechanistic understanding of the action of that gene in controlling fat synthesis and breakdown in the human fat cell— a mechanism that formed the initial framework for our subsequent work in calcium and dairy regulation of fat cell metabolism. Other key players who collaborated with me and helped develop that work include Dr. William Wilkison; Dr. Naima Moustaid Moussa, my colleague at the University of Tennessee; and two former graduate students who were instrumental in completing this work: Dr. Jung Han Kim (who is now my colleague at the University of Tennessee) and Dr. Bingzhong Xue.

When that "aha" moment occurred, moving from broad concept to experimentation and understanding was a highly collaborative effort. My chief collaborator in most of the initial research was my (then) graduate student, Dr. Hang Shi. Hang was initially quite the skeptic, and I think he plunged himself into these experiments to prove me wrong! Nonetheless, as the supporting data emerged from our experiments, his skepticism waned, and he emerged as a truly brilliant creative force. It was a true pleasure having Hang as a challenging collaborator in developing and testing these ideas in the laboratory. As these ideas continue to evolve, as they must even after the publication of this book, Dr. Xiaocun Sun and Teresa Sobhani, members of my current laboratory group, work with me in continuing to refine, develop, and test these concepts.

Of course, these concepts only become relevant as we translate them from laboratory to clinic. We have already acknowledged the wonderful staff members of the Nutrition and Metabolic Research Clinic at the University of Tennessee. In addition, I have been fortunate in these clinical trials to have two physicians who have worked with me in planning and conducting these studies: Dr. Warren Thompson and Dr. Peter Campbell.

Finally, this book has become a reality due to the persistence and talent of my coauthor, Bill, who first had the foresight to want to develop our concepts into this book and who has had the talent and patience to work with me in turning obtuse scientific concepts into something practical and useful.

Bill:

Michael, my always gracious coauthor, for his understanding and patience during the lengthy development of this project, and for the creativity, expertise, and insights that led him and his colleagues to the compelling scientific discoveries presented in *The Calcium Key.*

The friends and family members who provided me with much-needed emotional support during the intense period of writing this book: the incredibly kind Jan; Dr. Dan and Ms. Is; Michael B of DC; Mr. Rollo; Randall "the fan" Fitzgerald; cat-satisfied Suzie; and, most constantly and uniquely—because there is "no Friend greater"—my Spiritual Master and Divine Heart-Companion, Avatar Adi Da Samraj.

Introduction

Can We End the Overweight Epidemic?

It is a question that health and medical experts all over America think about—and try to find answers for—every day. One of those experts is Robert P. Heaney, M.D., an endocrinologist and professor of medicine at Creighton University in Omaha, Nebraska. Dr. Heaney has conducted dozens of scientific studies on osteoporosis, the bone-thinning disease. Recently, he analyzed the data on several hundred women he had studied, probing for an association between calcium intake and weight gain. (He instigated this research based on studies of calcium and fat cells that my colleagues and I had conducted at the University of Tennessee—studies that show a low-calcium diet causes weight gain and a high-calcium diet increases the rate of weight loss. I discuss those studies in detail in chapter 1.) Dr. Heaney wanted to quantify the impact on the obesity epidemic if everyone in the United States got the amount of calcium recommended by the government: 1300 milligrams (mg) daily for adolescents and young adults 9 to 18 years old; 1000 mg daily for adults 19 to 50; and 1200 mg daily for adults 51 and older. He summarized his results in the *Journal of Nutrition:* "The prevalence of obesity (or weight gain) could be reduced by 60 to 80% by the simple stratagem of ensuring population-wide calcium intake at the currently recommended levels."

Dr. Heaney's bold assertion is linked to the proven promise of *The Calcium Key:* any person who follows the Calcium Key Weight-Loss Plan can potentially double his or her body's ability to lose weight and fat.

It's important to point out that the Calcium Key Weight-Loss Plan (presented in practical detail in chapter 2) does a lot more than increase your intake of calcium. It delivers most of its calcium via dairy foods, which my studies show increase fat burning and decrease fat making and fat storage by 50% more than obtaining calcium from nondairy sources. It also emphasizes foods scientifically proven to satisfy your appetite and reduce hunger, which are crucial elements in any weight-loss plan. It recommends an easy-to-achieve level of calorie cutting, which is a must for any diet that is actually going to work. And it shows you how to burn calories with easy exercise and daily activities. I've included all of those features in the plan, because they're all necessary for successful weight loss.

I can understand if you want to turn now to chapters 1 and 2 and start learning about dairy's power to double your weight and fat loss. But before you read about the discovery of the calcium–fat connection, and the Calcium Key Weight-Loss Plan, you may want to keep reading this chapter, in order to better understand the overweight epidemic. An improved understanding of any problem is the key to solving it. So, to serve that purpose, I'd like to address and answer a couple of questions about the overweight epidemic.

Let's begin at the beginning: What is overweight?

The Three Faces of Fat: Overweight, Obesity, and Extreme Obesity

Scientists have categorized and labeled the levels of body fat. But they don't measure fat cells per pound. They use a measurement called BMI, or body mass index. Based on height and weight, BMI uses the following mathematical formula to assign a range of numbers to levels of fatness:

$$\text{weight in kilograms} \div \text{height in meters}^2,$$

or, in nonmetric terms:

$$\text{weight in pounds} \div \text{height in inches} \div \text{height in inches} \times 703.$$

Why use BMI? Because it's a simple, rapid, and inexpensive way to calculate body fat, and it's accurate.

According to the National Heart, Lung, and Blood Institute of the National Institutes of Health, the following are the BMI levels for adults for what scientists call underweight, normal weight, overweight, obesity, and extreme obesity:

Underweight	18.4 or less
Normal weight	18.5 to 24.9

Overweight	25 to 29.9
Obesity	30 to 39.9
Extreme obesity	40 or more

For example, if you're 5'6" and weigh 130 pounds, your BMI is 21, so your weight is normal (it's the level of body fat that poses the lowest risk of disease and death). At 5'6" and 155 pounds, your BMI is 25, so you're considered overweight. At 5'6" and 186 pounds, your BMI is 30, so you're officially obese. At 5'6" and 247 pounds, your BMI is 40, so you are extremely obese.

In a recent study published in the *Journal of the American Medical Association (JAMA)*, scientists from the National Center for Health Statistics at the Centers for Disease Control and Prevention (CDC) looked at data from the National Health and Nutrition Examination Survey (NHANES), an ongoing project that records the health and eating habits of thousands of Americans. They categorized a so-called representative sample of more than 4000 Americans into the above categories of weight. Their results indicated that 34% of adults aged 20 to 74 are overweight, 26% are obese, and 5% are extremely obese.

The *JAMA* article said that 65% of American adults have a BMI of 25 or more, 31% can be classified as obese, and 5% can be classified as extremely obese. Only about 35% of Americans are normal weight.

Any way you look at the numbers, you're looking at an epidemic of fatness. This epidemic isn't limited to adults. The same researchers looked at overweight among children and adolescents. (For kids, experts use a slightly different BMI formula that takes age into account.) They found the following percentages of kids were either overweight or at risk for overweight (very close to the overweight category): 21% of 2- to 5-year-olds, 30% of 6- to 11-year-olds, 30% of 12- to 19-year-olds.

The Causes of Overweight

Why is the overweight epidemic happening? What is the cause? It's clearly not genetic. Our genes take thousands of years to change, not a decade or two.

The cause of the overweight epidemic can be found in our environment. Specifically, we are experiencing a dramatic increase in the availability of calories and a dramatic decrease in calorie-burning activities.

Understanding how people gain weight is quite simple. I call it The Calorie Equation. It says that if you ingest more calories (energy) than you burn, you gain weight. If you ingest fewer calories than you burn, you lose weight. If you ingest the same amount of calories as you burn, you maintain weight.

The overweight epidemic is a result of North Americans ingesting more calories than they burn. Let's take a look at what's happened to our calorie intake from food and our calorie burning from daily activities and exercise.

① *More calories ingested:* Year by year, more calories have crept into our diet. Surveys show that from 1978 to 1996, the average daily calorie intake increased from 2239 to 2455 calories in men, and from 1534 to 1646 calories in women. The average increase for all Americans: 167 calories a day— a pace that could pile on 17 extra pounds of fat in a year!

② *From huge portions:* Food portions are preposterous. Candy bars are starting to look like crowbars. Soft drinks, once served in 6-ounce bottles, are routinely poured into 32- and even 64-ounce containers, delivering hundreds of extra calories.

One study found larger portions were being served at home. A typical home-cooked burger, for example, was 5.7 ounces in 1977. Now it's 8.4 ounces—an increase of 225 calories. Data from the U.S. Department of Agriculture show that America's per-person food production has risen by 400 calories a day since 1978.

③ *And more snacks:* We're not pigging out—we're cowing out. As a nation, we eat like cows, constantly grazing on high-calorie snack foods. A study from researchers at Harvard shows that Americans have doubled their calorie consumption from snacks since the 1980s.

④ *And frequent fast-food meals:* Fast is in—Americans now eat 25% of all their meals at fast-food restaurants—up from 10% in 1977. Fast food may be a good deal for your pocketbook, but it can be a bad deal for your waistline.

A large hamburger, supersize fries, and large soda add up to 1500 calories. The energy needs for a woman of average size are approximately 2000 calories a day; for a man, 2700. One typical fast-food meal provides 75% of a woman's necessary daily calories and 56% of a man's. So, it's not easy to stay slim on fast food.

There's nothing wrong with fast-food restaurants per se; it's possible to eat fast and well. Unfortunately, that's not what most people are doing.

⑤ *Fewer calories burned from regular exercise:* Only 14% of North Americans get regular, intense physical exercise. In fact, research shows that our level of physical activity hasn't changed from 1991 to 1998—even as our calorie consumption has gone up. A 200-pound person who is not cutting calories but who walks briskly for 1½ miles a day can lose more than a pound a month.

⑥ *Less opportunity for everyday calorie burning:* Labor-saving devices are everywhere. We don't wash dishes by hand; we use the dishwasher. We don't shovel snow; we use a snow blower. We don't walk up stairs; we ride the escalator or elevator. We don't wash the car; we drive to a carwash. We don't get up to change the channel; we use the remote control. We don't roll down the car window; we press a button. We don't push the lawnmower; we ride it. (Maybe soon we won't even be walking the dog, now that robot pets are increasingly popular.)

Does all that automation really make a difference in whether people gain weight? Definitely.

An hour of housework, for example, burns about 150 calories. If you burned 150 more calories a day than you do now, you would lose 10 pounds in 6 months, or 20 pounds in a year.

Do You Have Fat Disease?

Extra pounds mean extra risk of disease and death. The CDC compiled the following list of conditions and diseases you're more likely to get with a BMI over 25:

- High blood pressure
- High cholesterol
- Type II (non-insulin-dependent) diabetes
- Heart disease
- Stroke
- Gallstones
- Gout
- Osteoarthritis
- Sleep apnea
- Cancer (breast, prostate, and colon, among others)
- Pregnancy complications
- Poor female reproductive health (menstrual irregularities and infertility)
- Bladder-control problems
- Psychological disorders (depression, eating disorders, distorted body image, and low self-esteem)

The good news: losing about 5 to 10% of your body weight can dramatically lower your risk from heart disease, diabetes, and other killers.

Obviously, you'd like to lower your risk of death. And maybe you've tried many times to permanently lose 5 to 10% of your weight—and failed.

Failure is in your past. Success is your present—success with the Calcium Key Weight-Loss Plan.

A Way Out of the Overweight Epidemic

Surveys show that 75% of North Americans are either trying to lose weight or not gain weight. The statistics you read in this chapter show that few are succeeding. And so do other scientific findings. According to a review of 60 years of studies on weight loss published in *Obesity Review*, 85% of those who lose weight regain it.

Sure, you can follow the government's commonsense suggestions to exercise regularly, eat reasonable portions, and increase your consumption of low-calorie, nutrient-dense foods like fruits and vegetables. These elements are crucially important for weight loss. But is there something else you can and should do to lose weight? Is something missing? Is there a previously undiscovered and crucial element to weight loss that can dramatically increase your likelihood of diet success?

Since 1990, my colleagues and I at the Nutrition Department of the University of Tennessee have made a series of discoveries about how the body burns and stores fat. I think these findings will help our individual and collective ability to reverse the obesity epidemic.

We have discovered that dietary calcium plays a major role in controlling how fat cells work—how they make fat, burn fat, and store fat. We have discovered that adding calcium-rich dairy foods to the diet doubles the rate of weight loss and fat loss. We have discovered the Calcium Key—the way to unlock your fat cells to lose weight. Quickly. Permanently. Healthfully.

You've read about the overweight epidemic. You understand its dimensions; you understand that it causes not only discomfort but disease and death. You know about the problem. Now it's time to read about the solution.

The Remarkable, Life-Changing
Promise of the Calcium Key

What kind of changes can you expect if you follow the Calcium Key Weight-Loss Plan in this book?

Compared to a diet that only controls calories, breakthrough scientific studies show that the Calcium Key Weight-Loss Plan can

- Increase the amount of weight you lose by 70%
- Increase the amount of body fat you lose by 64%
- Help you lose 47% more fat from your belly
- Decrease the likelihood that you'll regain the weight you lost

These remarkable changes can happen because the Calcium Key Weight-Loss Plan transforms how your fat cells work. Your fat cells will make less fat, burn more fat, and store less fat. These are not wild claims. They are scientific facts proven in study after study conducted at my own laboratory and clinic at the University of Tennessee and by other researchers worldwide.

The key to unlocking your fat cells is getting the right number of servings a day of high-calcium dairy products and following the other suggestions of the Calcium Key Weight-Loss Plan.

Are you ready to be slim and healthy for the rest of your life? Read on.

PART I

THE MISSING LINK IN WEIGHT LOSS

1

Discovering the Calcium–Fat Connection

Susan's Story: 48 Pounds Lost

Susan is a foster parent who cooks and cares for four children. With the intense stress of her daily life, she found it extremely difficult to lose weight. But the 45-year-old didn't have any problem shedding pounds as soon as she went on the Calcium Key Weight-Loss Plan.

"This was the easiest, nondreading-it diet I've ever been on," she told me. Susan found the diet easy to understand and easy to follow. She could eat all the regular foods she normally ate, even fried chicken. She could cook for herself, her husband, and her kids at the same time, just as long as she counted her exchanges. When she felt hungry between meals, she would grab a carrot or fruit or other low-calorie but filling food. And she used fruit-flavored yogurt to satisfy her sweet tooth so that she didn't eat too much candy or cake.

Susan, who is 5'9", lost 48 pounds on the Calcium Key Weight-Loss Plan, going from 201 to 153 pounds. Susan had a lot of fun losing weight. Everybody at her church noticed how much weight she'd lost. They asked her whether she was on a diet. And she laughed and said, "No, I'm just eating right and drinking a lot more milk!"

Her husband is Susan's biggest supporter. Just about every day he looks at her and says, "Honey, you're looking *good.*"

Since grade school, you've been told that calcium is good for your teeth and your bones. You know that. Everybody knows that.

But what you may not know is that calcium is good for a lot more than a bright smile and a healthy skeleton. If you didn't have enough of this mineral circulating in your bloodstream, here's what would happen:

- Your heart wouldn't beat.
- Your blood wouldn't clot.
- Your hormones wouldn't send the chemical messages that regulate a wide range of metabolic functions in your body, from temperature to appetite to sleep.
- Your nerves wouldn't transmit electrical signals—you wouldn't move a muscle, digest food, or perform any action.

Calcium is so critical to your body's moment-to-moment functioning that when blood levels drop below the amount required by your cells, one of your body's possible responses is to steal calcium from its crystalline home in the bones. Sure, you can end up with osteoporosis, the bone-thinning disease. But you're still alive—and that's your body's first priority.

Calcium is a necessity for life, which is one of the reasons I've spent most of the 25 years of my scientific career studying this fascinating mineral. I wanted to know exactly how the body manages to retain or lose calcium. And I wanted to know exactly how this crucial nutrient functions in health and disease.

This chapter is the story of the quest for more knowledge about calcium—and better health for everyone. Step by step, year by year, this quest has led me and my fellow researchers to discover a role for calcium that neither we nor any other scientist ever expected to find: along with its other crucial functions within the cells of the body, calcium affects fat cells, regulating how much fat is made, how much fat is stored, and how much fat is burned.

In this chapter, I'll tell you about this discovery and all that it means for your quest for permanent weight loss. But first, I want you to understand the biochemical mechanisms by which calcium helps control weight. That way, when you begin to follow the recommendations of the Calcium Key Weight-Loss Plan, you won't have any doubts about the scientific efficacy of what you're doing. You'll know that the Calcium Key Weight-Loss Plan will work, because you'll have seen for yourself that study after published scientific study—over 40 in all—have proven that it works.

This is the story of the discovery of the missing link in weight loss: the story of calcium and fat cells, particularly of how high-calcium foods like dairy products can change the metabolism of fat cells, helping you to prevent weight gain or to shed extra pounds. The story begins with an investigation into an area seemingly unrelated to calcium and overweight (but that actually is directly connected): high blood pressure, or essential hypertension.

The Calcium Paradox

The first hint of a cause-and-effect relationship between calcium and high blood pressure came in the 1960s. Scientists discovered that people who drank water that contained a lot of calcium carbonate (hard water) had fewer heart attacks and strokes than people who drank water with very little calcium carbonate (soft water). High blood pressure is a risk factor for both of these diseases. Scientists asked themselves if calcium could be protecting people against high blood pressure.

Two Landmark Studies

In the early 1980s, David McCarron, M.D., professor of medicine at Oregon Health Sciences University in Portland, published two landmark papers on calcium and high blood pressure in *Science,* revolutionizing the way other scientists thought about this connection.

In a 1982 study, McCarron and a team of researchers looked at the dietary calcium intake of people with and without high blood pressure. They found that those with high blood pressure consumed an average of 668 milligrams (mg) of calcium, while those without the problem consumed 886 mg. "The data suggest that inadequate calcium intake may be a previously unrecognized factor in the development of hypertension," McCarron wrote.

In a 1984 study, McCarron and his colleagues analyzed nutritional data from the government's first massive survey of America's eating habits: the National Center for Health Statistics, Health and Nutrition Examination Survey, or NHANES-1. He looked at the link between the intake of 17 different nutrients and blood pressure levels in more than 10,000 men and women. The most significant link: calcium. The lower the level of calcium in the diet, the greater the risk of developing high blood pressure.

During the following two decades, dozens of other scientific studies confirmed the link between calcium and high blood pressure. They showed that many people can reduce hypertension by having a daily calcium intake of 1000 to 1500 mg. They also showed that calcium from food has about twice the pressure-lowering power as calcium from supplements. I'd like you to remember this important point.

Frank's Story: Losing Those Love Handles

Frank is a 47-year-old executive for a trucking company. His best experience of being on the Calcium Key Weight-Loss Plan was when his wife first noticed that he was losing weight around his midsection.

Frank's experience is similar to that of many men and women who go on the plan. Soon they (and their near-and-dear) start to experience a unique benefit: less abdominal fat. Love handles, stomach flab, a beer belly—whatever you want to call it—the plan can make it melt away.

Frank didn't only lose his gut. He lost 26 pounds, dropping from 220 to 194. Before being on the Calcium Key Weight-Loss Plan, Frank had never been able to lose weight. Once on the plan, he found it easy to shed pounds. One big change in his eating style that really helped was that instead of getting hungry and gorging himself at the next meal, he ate between-meal snacks of cheese or yogurt, satisfying his appetite.

His wife felt satisfied, too. For years, she'd been after Frank to do something about his weight. But the self-confessed procrastinator had never felt motivated to discipline his eating habits. With the Calcium Key Weight-Loss Plan, he didn't have to. He told me he just followed the exchange system and added dairy.

Frank felt kind of bad about himself when he started the plan. He was just too fat for his own liking. But now he feels good about himself. He lost weight—something he never thought he'd be able to do.

At the time McCarron's research appeared, I was an associate professor at Wayne State University in Detroit. And I was immediately interested in trying to discover the mechanism of calcium's effect on blood pressure, specifically how the nutrient worked to improve health. This task was complicated by the calcium paradox of essential hypertension.

The source of the paradox: at the same time that McCarron was discovering that a calcium-rich diet could protect against high blood pressure, doctors were writing millions of prescriptions for calcium channel blockers—drugs that treat high blood pressure by blocking the entrance of calcium into the cells. The drugs work because when calcium enters the smooth muscle cells of an artery, it causes the artery to constrict or narrow, raising blood pressure. Blocking calcium from entering the cells keeps the arteries wider and blood pressure normal.

How could both of these realities exist simultaneously? How could increasing calcium in the diet make blood pressure go down, while increasing calcium in the cells make blood pressure go up?

My colleagues and I—and other researchers, such as Lawrence Resnick, M.D., professor of medicine at the Hypertension Center at the New York

Weill Cornell Medical Center in New York City—knew that if we were to solve this paradox, we had to discover a mechanism whereby increasing calcium in the diet decreased calcium in the cells. Either we had to find a factor that pushed calcium into the cells—a factor removed by a high-calcium diet—or we had to find a factor that blocked calcium from entering the cells—a factor released by a high-calcium diet.

The Unexpected Role of the Hormone Calcitriol

Calcium plays a crucial role in regulating the core functions of the body. Needless to say, the body has evolved mechanisms to guarantee that blood calcium levels never drop too low. The main mechanism is hormonal. If calcium levels fall—if you eat a low-calcium diet, for example—the *parathyroids,* small glands on the surface of the thyroid gland, secrete *parathyroid hormone (PTH).* In turn, PTH triggers the release of another hormone, *calcitriol.*

Calcitriol helps your body make the best use of calcium. It increases absorption in the intestines, so you get the most calcium possible from food. And it increases reabsorption from the kidneys, so you lose as little as possible through excretion.

In our research, we focused on calcitriol as the factor that might be responsible for the calcium paradox. And in the laboratory, using animal models of human hypertension, we and other researchers found something we never expected to find. Calcitriol didn't only act on the cells of the intestines and the kidneys to help the body absorb and retain calcium. It also acted on the smooth muscle cells of the arteries, allowing calcium to move into these cells, thereby raising blood pressure. The calcium paradox of essential hypertension had been resolved. It turned out that

1. Low dietary levels of calcium cause an increase in the body's manufacture of calcitriol. Higher levels of calcitriol cause more calcium to enter the smooth muscle cells of the arteries. More calcium in these cells causes the arteries to narrow, raising blood pressure.
2. High dietary levels of calcium cause a decrease in the body's manufacture of calcitriol. Lower levels of calcitriol cause less calcium to enter the smooth muscle cells of the arteries. Less calcium in these cells keeps the arteries relaxed, maintaining normal blood pressure.

In the 1990s, this discovery about calcitriol and calcium levels in smooth muscle cells would play a crucial role in the scientific discovery of calcitriol and calcium levels in fat cells.

Studying a Salt-Sensitive Population

Low calcium intake isn't the only reason people get high blood pressure. Many different factors can cause it. That's why there are so many different types of drugs available to treat high blood pressure—each targets a different factor. My colleagues and I were interested in investigating several of these factors and discovering if calcium was the link between them.

For example, we were studying insulin resistance. In this problem, the hormone insulin is less effective than it should be in ushering blood sugar into cells; insulin resistance is often the first stage in the development of type II (adult-onset) diabetes. People who are insulin resistant also tend to be overweight, have higher than normal levels of the blood fat triglycerides, and have high blood pressure. This is a grouping of problems that Gerald Reaven, M.D., professor at Stanford University School of Medicine, has called syndrome X, which is also referred to as the insulin resistance syndrome and the metabolic syndrome. I wondered if there was a connection among all of the problems of the metabolic syndrome.

As part of our effort to answer this question, we conducted a study of African-American men with high blood pressure. African-Americans, like people over 60, are known to be salt-sensitive. In general, when they eat too much salt, their bodies excrete more calcium, which sparks an increase in PTH, increasing calcitriol and increasing blood pressure. For African-Americans and those over 60, calcium is often an excellent treatment for high blood pressure. Could it also treat insulin sensitivity?

In our study, we gave African-American men 2 cups of low-fat yogurt a day, increasing their daily calcium intake from 400 mg to 1000 mg. After a year, we had results.

On average, blood pressure fell and insulin resistance normalized. But there was a result we didn't expect: the men lost an average of 11 pounds of body fat.

I had no explanation for this result. In fact, it made no sense to me whatsoever. Why did they shed fat and gain muscle? They didn't eat fewer calories. They didn't exercise more. I decided it was just one of those stray observations that should go unpublished—the result of chance rather than any scientifically verifiable factor.

But even though I never published the result, that didn't stop me from talking to other scientists about it. And frequently researchers would tell me that they had conducted a study in which they also saw a direct relationship between dietary calcium and body fat—that is, higher calcium intake, lower fat—but because they couldn't explain the result, they didn't publish it.

It made me think that this wasn't just some random observation. There really was something going on. Little did I know that my colleagues and I had put together the first piece of the puzzle—the calcitriol connection. Or that I was about to have a lucky break—a seemingly random but very important scientific connection that would lead to the next step in discovering the missing link between calcium and fat.

The Obesity Gene

Scientists have developed a complex biological technology that enables them to clone the genes that contribute to obesity in mice. For years, researchers had speculated about the existence of these genes. They'd seen how mice from two different genetic strains could eat the same number of calories, with one genetic group staying thin and the other getting fat.

The point of these experiments wasn't to figure out how to help mice lose weight. Scientists knew that if genes determined overweight in mice, they probably played a role in determining overweight in people, too. If researchers could understand obesity genes, perhaps they could understand the complex biochemical processes that triggered obesity and target those processes with medications or nutritional changes.

The scientific challenge was to find the mice obesity genes and clone them—because with cloning, researchers could work with a gene. They could know its sequence of DNA, the code for making the proteins or enzymes that perform the functions in the cell. They could also make those proteins and put them into cells. They could look at the gene and the cells and the whole animal—and could really start to understand how the gene works in health and disease.

Fortunately for me, the first obesity gene in mice was cloned in 1992 by Rick Woychik, Ph.D., at Oak Ridge National Laboratory in Tennessee—just 30 miles down the road from where I was working in Knoxville as director of the University of Tennessee Nutrition Institute. Shortly after Woychik cloned the gene, I attended one of his presentations and talked to him afterward about a possible collaboration. He had discovered the gene; I wanted to work with him on discovering its mechanism because I had some intriguing ideas about what the gene does. Woychik agreed.

The name of the gene cloned by Woychik is *agouti*. When a mouse is born, *agouti* tells proteins to instruct biological pigments to color the mouse's hairs with a black tip, a band of yellow underneath it, and a black shaft. But a number of mutated or overexpressed genetic strains of *agouti* also influence a wide range of metabolic functions in a mouse—they cause mice to have a tendency to be overweight, insulin resistant, grow faster, and burn fewer calories than normal.

Mice with *agouti* mutations—so-called *transgenic mice*—aren't much different than a person with a weight problem. Interestingly enough, the *agouti* gene is also expressed in human fat tissue; the structure of *agouti* in humans and in mice is about 80% the same. We may not like to admit it, but on the genetic level mice and people aren't all that different, which is why studying mouse models of health and disease can help us understand how human bodies work.

Agouti = More Calcium = Bigger Fat Cells

My colleagues and I focused intensively on *agouti,* publishing 20 scientific studies on the gene's mechanism from 1992 to 2000. One of the first things we discovered was that *agouti* plays a role in the movement of calcium into the cell—that mice with *agouti* mutations have more *intracellular* calcium (within the cell) than normal mice. Another study showed that the more *agouti,* the higher the levels of calcium in the cell and the higher the animal's body weight.

Our research was indicating a direct relationship between intracellular calcium and overweight in these animals. Logically, we continued to focus on *agouti,* calcium, and fat cells—both mouse fat cells and human fat cells. We discovered that *agouti* causes an increase in calcium in human fat cells, which turns on a system for making more fat and turns off a system for breaking down fat.

On Fat and Your Genes

To better understand what these findings mean in terms of your ability to lose weight, let's take a short break from the story of the discovery of the calcium–fat connection and just talk about fat.

People used to think of bone as a static structure, like a girder holding up your body. Now they understand that bone is living, changing tissue. Similarly, fat is not just a blob attached to the body. It's made up of dynamic cells that are alive and active. These cells make fat, store fat, break down or burn fat, and make it available to the rest of the body as energy.

We discovered that increasing calcium in fat cells tilts the living processes toward fat storage and away from fat breakdown. Increasing calcium in fat cells tells the cells to become more efficient. Efficiency was crucial for our hunter-gatherer forebears. They never knew where their next meal was coming from, so the primitive human body evolved mechanisms to efficiently store food as energy and to be stingy about releasing that energy. But in our postindustrial society, where excess is the problem rather than scarcity, efficiency has turned out to be a lousy evolutionary adaptation. For optimum weight loss, we want to waste energy.

If we want to waste energy, we've got to reduce the amount of calcium in fat cells. Our research has shown that reducing calcium in fat cells causes the cells to make less fat and break down more fat.

Agouti has been a flashlight—a tool to light the way toward what is important in the study of obesity. But genes aren't what's broken in people who are overweight. It's not our genes that have shifted in the last generation as overweight has become epidemic; it's our environment. A changing environment—more available calories and fewer opportunities for calorie-burning activity—has acted upon our susceptible genes. If we didn't have those susceptible genes, perhaps we could have resisted the environmental changes. Our problem is not genetic: it's finding the right medical or nutritional interventions to help our bodies resist the changing environment. This was the next step in our research.

Preventing Bigger, Fatter Fat Cells

One of the discoveries that allowed us to move beyond *agouti* was identifying the effect of calcium on a protein in fat cells called *fatty acid synthase (FAS)*. We found that calcium stimulates a gene to make more FAS and that FAS plays a key role in the creation of triglycerides in fat cells. In addition, we found that another protein, the sulfonylurea receptor, plays a role in letting calcium into and out of the fat cell.

In animal experiments, we tried to influence these calcium-controlling proteins with medications. In one study, we gave mice high doses of nifedipine, a drug that keeps calcium out of the cells. After receiving the drug, FAS activity in the mice decreased by 74%, and there was an 18% decrease in body fat. We had proven that calcium levels in fat cells can be reduced by medications, with a subsequent reduction in overall fat. We patented those two proteins as sites for the pharmacological treatment of obesity. (The development of those drugs is many years in the future.)

With those results in hand, I asked myself if we could do the same thing nutritionally—if we could somehow use diet to reduce calcium in fat cells and thereby promote smaller, thinner fat cells.

My Calcium "Aha!"

I remembered the data on the African-American men who had increased their levels of dietary calcium and lost 11 pounds of fat in 1 year—the data

I had never published because I couldn't figure out why calcium reduced fat levels.

Could the calcium paradox of essential hypertension also be the calcium paradox of obesity? Could high levels of dietary calcium result in low levels of calcium in fat cells by the same mechanism that high levels of dietary calcium result in low levels of calcium in smooth muscle cells of the arteries?

I wondered if low dietary levels of calcium caused an increase in the body's manufacture of calcitriol, higher levels of calcitriol caused more calcium to enter fat cells, and more calcium in fat cells caused them to store more fat and burn less fat. Conversely, if high dietary levels of calcium caused a decrease in the body's manufacture of calcitriol, lower levels of calcitriol caused less calcium to enter fat cells, and less calcium in fat cells allowed them to store less fat and burn more fat. We immediately started to conduct new studies.

Calcitriol: Friendly to Fat

In the laboratory, we isolated human fat cells in petri dishes and put calcitriol on them. The results were astonishing.

Calcitriol triggered large increases in the amount of calcium in the cells—in fact, the amount of calcium tripled. As calcium went up, fat storage in the cells increased and fat burning decreased.

We had proved a direct connection between the hormone calcitriol, calcium levels in fat cells, and how fat cells function. We had proved that calcitriol—which we generally think of as regulating the absorption of calcium and playing a key role in bone metabolism—was crucial for regulating the function of fat cells. And we knew there was only one scientifically proven way to suppress this hormone: by increasing the intake of dietary calcium. The next step was to see if a high-calcium diet could, in fact, affect not only the fat cells, but patterns of weight gain and weight loss. To do that, we studied transgenic mice.

High-Fat, High-Sugar, High-Calcium Experimental Diets

Our first study of mice was published in the June 2000 issue of the *FASEB Journal*. We separated mice into four different dietary groups. Group 1 ate a low-calcium (0.4% of the total diet), high-fat, high-sugar diet. Group 2 ate the same diet—the same number of calories—but we added calcium in supplemental form, increasing calcium levels to 1.2% of the diet. Group 3 ate a similar high-fat, high-sugar diet, but we replaced 25% of the protein in the diet with nonfat dry milk, putting calcium levels at 1.2%. Group 4 also ate a similar diet, but we replaced 50% of the protein with nonfat dry milk, increasing calcium to 2.4%.

After 6 weeks of feeding the mice, we measured the overall weight gain of each animal and the total mass of fat in their fat pads, four areas of fat accumulation in mice. The results were remarkable.

Obviously, all four of the groups gained weight—these mice were eating a lot of calories. Over the 6 weeks of the study, Group 1 had a weight gain of 24%. But the other three groups had a much smaller weight gain. In Group 2 (calcium supplement), the weight gain was 26% less than Group 1. In Group 3 (25% dairy), the weight gain was 29% less than Group 1. In Group 4 (50% dairy), the weight gain was 36% less than Group 1. The huge differences occurred in spite of there being no difference in calorie levels.

The mice that ate calcium-enriched diets also had higher core temperatures—that is, a higher rate of metabolism. Clearly, the mice were burning more fat and storing less. When we looked at the fat cells of the mice getting high-calcium diets, we found fat burning increased approximately 3- to 5-fold, with higher levels of fat burning sparked by the high-dairy rather than the calcium-supplement diet.

The results held up when we looked at the actual fat in the fat pads of the mice: we found 36% less fat in the calcium-fed mice as compared to the Group 1 mice not getting calcium. Needless to say, my colleagues and I thought these results were very interesting. We asked ourselves if there was a similar effect in humans—if adding calcium helped people not get fat.

High-Calcium Diets Keep You Thin

We turned to the same source of data that Dr. McCarron used to figure out that lower calcium intake translates into higher blood pressure: the most recent National Health and Nutrition Examination Survey, or NHANES-III.

We used statistical methods to control for other variables in the data, such as calorie intake, physical activity, age, race, and ethnicity. We separated all the participants into four levels of calcium intake and assigned each of them a number according to the relative risk of being the fattest. These were the results:

- If the average calcium intake was very low—an average of 255 mg a day, or about a half serving of dairy—the person had a relative risk of 1. He or she was going to be among the fattest.
- If the average calcium intake was 488 mg a day—about 1 serving of dairy—the relative risk was .75. The person had 25% less chance of being among the fattest.

- If the average calcium intake was 773 mg a day—about 2 servings of dairy—the relative risk was .40. The person had 60% less chance of being among the fattest.
- And if the person was among the few who met or exceeded the recommended levels of calcium—an average of 1346 mg a day, or 3 to 3½ servings of dairy—the relative risk was .16. He or she had 84% less chance of being among the fattest.

Wouldn't you like to cut your chances of being fat by 84% simply by eating more calcium-rich foods every day?

Calcium for Weight Loss

All of the research up to this point shows that calcium can help prevent weight gain. But what you probably want to hear about is if calcium can help you lose weight.

The Fat Mice Lost Weight When They Got Calcium

We returned to the laboratory and conducted another experiment with mice. First, we fed a group of mice a high-fat, high-sugar, low-calcium diet. They got fat. In 6 weeks, they had a 30% increase in weight, and their body fat level doubled.

Then we separated the mice into five groups. They all ate the same high-fat, high-sugar diet, but Group 1 got to eat all they wanted of the high-fat, high-sugar, low-calcium diet. Group 2 got the same diet but only 70% of the calories. We called this the calorie-restricted group. Group 3 was also calorie restricted to 70%, but calcium was added to their diet, as if they were taking a nutritional supplement. We called this the high-calcium group. Group 4 had a similar level of calorie restriction and calcium, but they got their calcium from nonfat dry milk, with 25% of protein replaced by milk. We called this the medium-dairy group. Group 5 was similar in calorie restriction and calcium but got 50% of protein replaced by milk. We called this the high-dairy group.

- The calorie-restricted group lost 11% of their weight. But the high-calcium group lost 19%, the medium-dairy group lost 25%, and the high-dairy group lost 29%.
- The calorie-restricted group had an 8% decrease in their fat pad mass. But fat levels in the high-calcium group decreased 42%; the medium-dairy group, 60%; and the high-dairy group, 69%.

- We also measured fat breakdown in fat cells. There was no increase in fat breakdown in the calorie-restricted group. The high-calcium group had a 77% increase; the medium-dairy and high-dairy groups had a 155% increase.
- We measured fat production in the fat cells, or what scientists call *fat synthesis*. The high-calcium group had a 35% decrease in fat synthesis; the medium-dairy group, 63%; the high-dairy group, 62%.
- Additionally, we looked at *core temperature*—that is, the metabolism of the mice. The high-calcium, medium-dairy, and high-dairy diets all had increased core temperatures, indicating the animals were wasting a lot more energy.

This study made it obvious that calcium not only prevents weight gain but also promotes weight loss. High-calcium diets stop calcium from entering the fat cells. The result: less fat is formed, less fat is stored, and more fat is burned. Body fat goes down, and so does weight. The study also made it obvious that more isn't better when it comes to adding dairy to the diet—the medium- and high-dairy groups lost almost the same amount of weight.

Calcium from Dairy Is More Effective Than Calcium Supplements

As you no doubt noticed, there was a big difference in this study between the effect of calcium in supplemental form and the effect of dairy. Overall, our research shows that dairy is 50 to 65% more effective than calcium supplementation in stopping fat storage and triggering fat breakdown. Why?

Scientifically speaking, I don't have the answer. It's not absorption; calcium in supplemental form and calcium from dairy are absorbed similarly. To date, there's been very little research into the exact mechanisms as to why dairy affects fat cells more powerfully than supplemental calcium. But I think there's a likely explanation.

You can't assume that if you use a supplement to get the primary nutrient in a food, you'll get the same benefit as if you ate the food. This nutritional perspective has been proven by two decades of research into *phytonutrients*—the various components of plants that aren't vitamins or minerals but are crucial to your health. We know, for example, that citrus fruits deliver more than vitamin C and carrots more than vitamin A. They also deliver anticancer and heart-protecting phytonutrients, like carotenoids, flavonoids, and lycopene.

The same is true of dairy. It contains calcium and a host of other biologically active compounds. For example, it contains an angiotensin-converting enzyme (ACE) inhibitor—a biochemical that helps prevent the narrowing of blood vessels and high blood pressure. It is used in drugs to treat hypertension. Knowing this, should you take a calcium supplement and an ACE inhibitor to replicate the benefits of eating dairy foods? Would they work together the same way as they do in dairy? Probably not. You would probably be missing other key compounds.

I'm not saying that attempting to isolate the components of dairy that aid weight loss isn't an important and necessary scientific endeavor; it is. Discovering these components will help us understand the new and exciting reality of dairy's power to transform fat cells. In fact, my colleagues and I at the University of Tennessee as well as many other scientists have begun to speculate about several of these factors.

One such factor is the ACE inhibitors we just discussed. They're found in whey, a dairy protein. New discoveries show that fat-making mechanisms in fat cells are regulated in part by angiotensin—the very chemical that ACE inhibitors block. Whey protein is also a rich source of leucine, an amino acid. Recent research reveals that leucine may increase the ability of muscle to burn fat.

But we can't simply reduce dairy to calcium, ACE inhibitors, and leucine. In nutrition, trying to understand a food's effect by understanding one or two of its parts doesn't work. A food is a complex mixture of known and unknown components. And there is a cooperation among the components of food that cannot be reproduced in a nutritional supplement. That's why the emphasis in this book on calcium and weight loss is on calcium from food—and primarily from low-fat dairy food, nature's richest source of the mineral.

How much dairy do you need? My colleagues and I have concluded from our study that between 1200 and 1600 mg of calcium a day from dairy is optimal for weight loss, or 3 to 4 servings of dairy a day. (In the Calcium Key Weight-Loss Plan, dairy supplies 900 to 1200 mg of the calcium; the rest is supplied by other foods.) In chapter 2, you'll find all the information you need to use dairy foods to lose weight.

Other Scientists Confirm Our Weight Loss Findings in People

Many other scientists began to publish studies on people that confirmed our findings on calcium and weight loss in mice. Writing in the *Journal of the American College of Nutrition*, researchers at Purdue University conducted a 2-year study of 54 women, ages 18 to 31, in which they measured the effect of regular exercise on bone mass. The women also filled out dietary records during the study, and the researchers recorded their weight, body fat, and muscle mass over the 2 years.

The researchers analyzed their data and discovered that the best predictor of weight and fat was calcium intake from dairy products. Women on low-calcium diets gained weight; women on high-calcium diets lost weight. These results were independent of whether the women were exercising or not.

However, these results did not hold up when women ate approximately 1900 or more calories per day. Calcium is not magic. If you ingest too many calories, you'll gain weight no matter what else you do. But if you eat the appropriate level of calories, calcium can make a huge difference in your effort to shed pounds.

Researchers at the Osteoporosis Research Center at Creighton University in Nebraska were intrigued by the calcium/weight-loss connection, so they reexamined their data from five studies on calcium and bone density. Dividing women into low- and high-calcium intake groups, they found women with low intake were 2¼ times more likely to be overweight than women with high intake. And here's an even more impressive statistic: women who got 1000 mg less calcium than their counterparts were on average 18 pounds heavier.

Writing in the *Journal of Clinical Endocrinology and Metabolism*, the authors of the study theorized that the evolutionary reason that calcium and weight are linked is that the primitive human diet was rich in calcium, with levels 2 to 4 times higher than what we ingest today. Genetically the body reads a lack of calcium as a food shortage, revving up cellular systems for fat production and shutting off systems for fat breakdown. The authors conclude, "Today, with calcium intake disconnected from energy [calorie] intake, the primitive energy-conserving response predisposes to weight gain."

But by getting enough calcium in your diet, you can be predisposed to weight loss!

My colleagues in the Nutritional Department at the University of Tennessee studied 53 children as they grew from preschool to school age. In the *International Journal of Obesity*, the researchers wrote that the strongest predictor of body fat among the children was calcium from dairy products. Children with higher intakes of dairy products had lower levels of body fat.

From 1985 to 1996, researchers from institutions around the world, including Harvard Medical School, studied 3000 people ages 18 to 30 in the Coronary Artery Risk Development in Young Adults (CARDIA) study. They were investigating the development of a health problem that we call metabolic syndrome, which they call insulin-resistance syndrome (IRS), and which is often called syndrome X—a potentially deadly combination of overweight, high blood sugar, high blood pressure, high triglycerides, and low levels of the good cholesterol HDL.

Writing in the *Journal of the American Medical Association*, the researchers reported that every time dairy products were eaten, the odds of being overweight went down—a 20% lower risk for each daily intake of a dairy food like milk, yogurt, or cheese. People who ate 3 servings of dairy a day had a 60% lower risk of being overweight.

But they also found that overweight people who consumed the most dairy—35 or more servings a week—were 71% less likely to develop IRS than people who consumed 10 or less servings per week. They concluded, "Dietary patterns characterized by increased dairy consumption may protect overweight individuals from the development of obesity and the insulin resistance syndrome, which are key risk factors for type II diabetes and cardiovascular disease."

In 2003, Robert Heaney, M.D., a scientist from Creighton University who coauthored the study showing that a calcium shortage of 1000 mg a day translates into 18 additional pounds of weight, decided to reanalyze his data. His goal was to calculate the effect that increasing calcium intake to recommended levels would have on the weight of the entire population of women. His startling conclusion: "The data presented in this analysis suggest that the prevalence of obesity (or weight gain) in women could be reduced by 60–80% by the simple stratagem of ensuring population-wide calcium intake at the currently recommended levels."

The government's recommended daily intake for calcium is 1300 mg for adolescents and young adults 9 to 18 years old, 1000 mg for adults 19 to 50, and 1200 mg for adults 51 and older. These amounts are easily met by the level of calcium in the Calcium Key Weight-Loss Plan.

My Own Research on People: Spectacular Results

The next study that I'll discuss is particularly close to my heart—because I led the team of researchers from the University of Tennessee who conducted it. In some ways, it represents the culmination of all the research in this chapter.

For the study, we put 32 overweight people on a balanced but restricted diet for 6 months, reducing their daily food intake by 500 calories. As the study started, we divided them into three groups.

The control group—the group against which the other groups were measured—received a low-calcium diet, with at most 1 serving of dairy a day, for a daily total of 400 to 500 mg of dietary calcium.

The second group received the same type of diet, along with an 800 mg supplement of calcium, to bring their calcium intake to 1200 to 1300 mg a day. This was the high-calcium group.

The third group got 3 servings of low-fat dairy a day, for a total of 1200 to 1300 mg of daily calcium. This was the high-dairy group.

At the beginning of the study, we measured the participants' weight, body fat, and waist size. We also used a special technique to measure the loss of abdominal fat compared to other parts of the body. When they started the study, our dieters were definitely overweight. They had a body mass index ranging from 30 to around 40, and they were eating a low-calcium diet of 500 to 600 mg a day.

Over the next 6 months, the control group lost approximately 6% of their total weight. In contrast, the high-calcium group lost almost 7.5% of their total weight—statistically, a 26% better showing than the control group. And the high-dairy group lost 11% of their total weight, for a 70% statistical improvement over the control group.

Fat loss was just as impressive. The control group lost 9% of their body fat. The folks from the high-calcium group lost 38% more fat than the control group. And the high-dairy group lost 64% more fat than the control group.

When we measured fat loss from the abdomen—the type of fat that puts you at the greatest risk for high blood pressure, high cholesterol and triglycerides, and insulin resistance, or metabolic syndrome—we found the control group lost 19% of their fat from the abdomen; the high-calcium group, 50%; and the high-dairy group, 66%. For the millions of women who are trying to tighten their tummies and the millions of men who are trying to lose their love handles, these unexpected results are really good news.

Patricia's Story: The Doctor Who Cured Herself of Overweight

Patricia, a 40-year-old physician, had mastered challenge after challenge as she became a pulmonary surgeon. She had the smarts, energy, and willpower to accomplish whatever she wanted—except losing weight.

Over the years, Patricia had been on many different diets. About 18 months ago, she tried a popular high-protein, low-carbohydrate diet, and she lost some weight. But she found she couldn't keep eating the way the diet said to eat. And just like with every other diet she'd ever tried, she eventually regained the weight she lost, and then some.

Patricia saw a notice for one of our studies posted on a bulletin board near the operating room where she worked. She decided to give weight loss one more try. She found there was a big difference between the Calcium Key Weight-Loss Plan and all the other diets she'd been on. She quickly discovered the plan was nutritionally well balanced, easy to follow, and a lot more effective.

Patricia started the Calcium Key Weight-Loss Plan at 175 pounds. Today, about a year later, she weighs 137 pounds. Her dress size went from a 16 to an 8. Even her blood pressure went down, from 130/90 to 110/70. She felt healthy when she was overweight, but she feels *really* healthy now.

Patricia says there are many reasons that the plan worked when all the other diets she tried hadn't. She never had to keep a tally of calories in her head but instead developed an easy routine of knowing how many exchanges she'd already had that day and how many more she had left. The Calcium Key Exchange System gave her much more flexibility than other diets, especially when she ate out. And she found the diet to be nutritious and sensible—nothing like the unbalanced, crazy diets she had tried in the past.

To Patricia, the best thing about the plan is how good it has made her feel inside and out. Her permanent weight loss has given her a real emotional boost. She feels gratified by her success and has much more self-confidence. She particularly enjoyed the positive feedback she got from family, friends, and coworkers as she lost weight. When she would run into people she hadn't seen her for a few weeks, they would almost always comment on how much *more* weight she'd lost.

The Calcium Key Weight-Loss Plan also helped Patricia's family. Her healthy style of eating provided a good role model for her 7-year-old son. Seeing her make healthy choices, he decided to do the same—and now he even prefers a salad to french fries. Her hope is that her son will never have to go on a diet because he'll never be overweight.

When a scientific study produces a positive result, one of the next things a scientist does is conduct the study again. By reproducing the result, evidence shows that the result is factual rather than accidental.

My colleagues and I recently conducted a study on dairy and weight loss similar to the one I just told you about. We reported the study at the yearly meeting of the Federation of American Societies for Experimental Biology.

We put people on a calorie-restricted diet and divided them into two groups. One group got 400 to 500 mg of dietary calcium a day from nondairy sources. The other group got 1100 mg of calcium a day, most of it from three 6-ounce servings of low-fat yogurt.

The study lasted for 12 weeks. Both groups lost weight and fat. But compared to the nondairy group, the yogurt group had 22% greater weight loss, 66% greater fat loss, and 81% greater abdominal fat loss.

Before the yogurt study, my colleagues and I conducted a study to see what effect dairy might have on overweight people who don't go on a diet. We reported the results at the annual convention of the American Heart Association.

In the study, 34 overweight but otherwise healthy African-American men and women were put on a special (but very simple) food regimen for 6 months. They ate either a low-calcium, low-dairy diet (less than 1 serving of dairy a day) or a high-calcium, high-dairy diet (3 servings of dairy a day). But neither group cut calories. The high-dairy group simply substituted calories from dairy for other calories that were in their diets. Nor did they change the levels of fat, protein, or carbohydrates.

The high-dairy group had a 26.5% increase in levels of glycerol, a chemical constituent of fat that shows up in the blood when the body breaks down fat. The low-dairy group didn't have a similar increase. But more importantly, the high-dairy group had a 5.4% decrease in total body fat, a 4.6% decrease in abdominal fat, and a 2.2% increase in lean body mass. The low-dairy group had no significant changes in any of these areas.

Without calorie restriction, without changing their diet in any way whatsoever, except to add dairy but not increase calories, the people in this study who ate 3 servings a day of dairy lost fat and gained muscle! That's pretty amazing.

There were other positive changes in the high-dairy group. They had an average decrease of 14% in insulin levels. That means their bodies were probably less insulin resistant. If someone is insulin resistant, the hormone insulin is less than optimally effective in moving blood sugar into the cells, and this condition is often a prelude to diabetes.

The high-dairy group also had a significant reduction in blood pressure: 6.8 points systolic (the upper measurement in a blood pressure reading). Most medications only reduce systolic pressure by about 12 points. Thus, overweight people who don't want to subtract calories can lose fat, build muscle, and get healthier, just by adding dairy.

Dairy May Stop the Weight from Coming Back

My studies show that dairy can help stop you from gaining weight. And they show that dairy more than doubles the rate at which you can lose weight and fat. But the fact remains that 85% of people who lose weight regain it. Can dairy actually help you keep weight off after you've lost it?

One of my newest studies also reported at the annual meeting of the Federation of American Societies for Experimental Biology shows the answer may be yes. A qualified yes, because the study was on mice. Even as this book was being written, I was conducting the same study on people, but I didn't have the results in time to include here. However, that doesn't mean what you're about to read won't give you new hope for permanent weight-loss success.

Once again, my colleagues and I experimented with *agouti* mice—mice that are genetically similar to overweight people. First, we fed all the mice a high-fat, high-sugar diet—and they all got fat. Next, we fed them a calorie-restricted, high-calcium diet—and they all lost weight. Then we divided them into three groups. All three groups were allowed to eat as much as they wanted. Group 1, however, was put on a low-calcium diet. Group 2 was put on a high-calcium diet, with the calcium from a food fortified with calcium carbonate. Group 3 was put on a high-dairy diet, with the same level of calcium intake as Group 2, but the calcium was from milk or yogurt. The mice ate those diets for 6 weeks.

The mice on the low-calcium diet regained all their weight. But the high-calcium and high-dairy diets prevented 53% of weight regain, which was astounding, because *agouti* mice allowed to eat all they want always get fat, just like Group 1 did. The high-calcium diet also prevented 55% of the fat regain while the high-dairy diet prevented 85% of the fat regain!

The study also confirmed some of what we already know about how dairy affects fat cells. The high-dairy diet increased fat burning by 271% and decreased FAS by 81%.

Can we expect the same results in people? The most that can be said at this point is that our previous studies show dairy doubles weight loss in mice and people, and hopefully the results of this study will be duplicated in people.

The story of the link between dairy foods and weight loss is not over. In fact, it's just beginning. We'll do more studies on people, as will other researchers. We'll continue to investigate the mechanisms of how calcium works in fat cells, seeking to refine our knowledge. We'll try to discover factors in dairy other than calcium that contribute to weight loss.

But, as you've read in this chapter, the moral of this story of discovering the missing link in weight loss couldn't be clearer: increasing dietary calcium from dairy products can help you lose weight. Specifically, it can more than double your rate of weight loss—70% more than if you merely restricted calories; more than double your rate of fat loss—64% more than if you merely restricted calories; and triple the rate of fat loss from your abdominal area. Next, we'll show you how to do just that.

PART II

THE CALCIUM KEY WEIGHT-LOSS PLAN

2

Unlocking Your Fat Cells
How to Use Dairy to Lose Weight

IT'S IMPORTANT TO EMPHASIZE that the Calcium Key Weight-Loss Plan is based on a new and revolutionary scientific understanding of the mechanisms of fat—scientifically proven discoveries about how fat is stored and burned, how it accumulates, and how it can dissolve. Among diet books, *The Calcium Key* is scientifically unique. It doesn't tout an unproven theory, like many other books on weight loss. It doesn't promote a diet that's never been clinically tested in rigorous, controlled research. It doesn't ask readers to believe the authors are misunderstood nutritional geniuses whose brilliant ideas will be accepted by scientists in the future. It is a weight-loss program with scientific studies that support its efficacy. These studies have been and continue to be replicated by top researchers all over the world. The Calcium Key is a new, unique, and simple way to lose weight that has been discovered in one of the world's leading nutritional centers and has been scientifically verified at the highest levels of international research.

But even though these discoveries have appeared in scientific journals and are summarized by statistical results, they were made by studying people. Real people with real weight problems.

And every person who wants to lose weight needs coaching—well-informed, proven advice about what to do and what not do to maximize the success of their efforts to shed pounds. In this chapter, you'll discover

- Why being aware of calories is an important part of the process of losing weight, but keeping an exact count isn't necessary (and can even be counterproductive).
- Why losing weight gradually is the best way to lose weight permanently, and losing weight as quickly as you can is a setup for long-term failure.

- How eating large amounts of nutrient-dense, calorie-moderate foods keeps your appetite satisfied as you lose weight. Yes, eating lots of food as you lose weight is possible, even necessary.
- How to use the glycemic index—a measure of how quickly carbohydrates turn into blood sugar in the body—to control hunger and keep fatigue at bay. You'll also learn that not all carbohydrates are the same: some help with weight loss and some hinder it.
- Why 35% of the calories in the Calcium Key Weight-Loss Plan are from fat and why low-fat diets are probably a prescription for weight-loss failure.

Be Calorie Conscious

That forerunner of potential pounds . . . those dictatorial data that threaten to punish you if you don't obey . . . that mealtime measurement some diet doctors say you have to count as carefully as an accountant. Who's right and who's wrong? Are calories a crucial factor in losing weight or aren't they? Here's an introductory and very brief course in weight-loss success.

Calories 101

A calorie is a unit of energy. We think of calories when we think of food, but scientists can use them to measure anything that contains energy. For example, the calories in one piece of cherry cheesecake could power a 60-watt lightbulb for 90 minutes. Sorry to say, there's no technology available to hook you up to your home's electrical system after dessert so that you can literally burn off that cheesecake.

You burn calories doing anything—even just sitting and reading this book. That's because right now your heart is burning calories so that it can beat, your lungs are burning calories so that you can breathe, your digestive tract is burning calories so that it can process the last meal you ate, and your brain is burning calories so that it can make sense of this sentence. The number of calories you burn while your body is at rest is called your *resting metabolic rate* and accounts for about 60 to 70% of the calories you burn a day.

If you were sitting in a boat fishing, you'd be burning about 2.4 calories a minute, but if you were spending a minute sitting and feeding a baby, you would burn about 3 calories; calorie burning increases to 3.4 per minute if you walk the dog and to 4 calories if you start raking leaves when you get back from your walk.

The foods that supply the fuel for these tasks—the carbohydrates, proteins, and fats in your daily diet—are also measured in calories. A gram (about 1/30 of an ounce) of carbohydrate or protein is 4 calories. A gram of fat is 9 calories.

Your body always stores extra calories as fat. A pound of body fat contains 3500 calories. A 40-year-old woman who is 5'6", weighs 165 pounds, and doesn't exercise burns about 2000 calories a day. If she cuts her daily intake of calories to 1500, she still burns 2000 a day, including 500 calories from her stored fat. During 1 week of eating 1500 calories, her body would burn an extra 3500 calories, or 1 pound of fat.

Now let's look at a 40-year-old man who is 5'9", weighs 160 pounds, and who doesn't exercise. He needs about 2500 calories a day to maintain his weight. If he gets that amount of calories in his diet and he starts walking an hour a day at a brisk pace, he'll burn an additional 250 calories. If he does that for a week, he'll burn 1750 calories, or a half pound of fat.

There is nothing mysterious about calories and weight. In the body, they are used for fuel or they are stored as fat. The role of calories in weight loss or weight gain is straightforward.

- If you take in more calories than you burn, you will gain weight.
- If you burn more calories than you take in, you will lose weight.
- If you take in the same amount of calories as you burn, you will maintain your weight.

You can, however, change how efficiently you burn calories. To lose weight, you want your fat cells to be inefficient. You want your body to waste more calories as heat and store fewer as fat. The studies my colleagues and I conducted at the University of Tennessee show that adding dairy to your diet does just that: dairy changes the way your fat cells work, making them more inefficient, so you store less fat and burn more calories. In fact, when you go on the Calcium Key Weight-Loss Plan—when you cut calories a little bit, increase exercise and daily activities a little bit, and add 3 to 4 servings of dairy foods to your diet—you can increase the rate at which you lose fat compared to a person who is only cutting calories and/or exercising more. The people who participated in our studies lost an average of 70% more fat.

But even if you add dairy to your diet, you can't ignore calories. If you want to lose weight, you will have to burn the calories stored in your body as fat by cutting some calories from your daily diet, including a little more exercise and activity in your daily life, and following the Calcium Key Weight-Loss Plan.

Dairy Is the Key to Weight Loss If You Don't Overdo the Calories

One study shows how a diet that's too high in calories can neutralize the Calcium Key Weight-Loss Plan. The 2-year study conducted at Purdue University looked at 54 women ages 18 to 31. Researchers found that the best indicator of weight loss was calcium intake from dairy products. Those who got high levels of calcium from dairy lost weight. Those who got low levels didn't.

But the researchers also found that if a woman's diet exceeded 1900 calories a day, calcium intake made no difference. Extra calcium couldn't help people who were getting extra calories. Dairy foods are not magic. If you ingest too many calories, you'll gain weight no matter what else you eat. But if you don't overdo it on calories, dairy foods can make a huge difference in your body's ability to shed pounds.

Dairy works by affecting what happens to calories in your body. You take in energy in the form of calories, utilizing some, wasting some, and storing the rest in the form of fat. A diet with 3 to 4 servings of dairy increases fat burning, ensuring the body expends the maximum number of calories. But only if you control your overall calorie intake.

Being Calorie Conscious = Weight-Loss Success

Scientific evidence shows that extra calories in the diet are a main cause of overweight. It also shows that calorie control can help solve the problem.

Unfortunately, only 21% of dieters do count calories, says a study in the *Journal of the American Medical Association*. Most people who want to lose weight prefer fad diets, says the study. Those diets work in the short term not because of their unique approach but because they restrict calories.

"All fad diets work in the same way—by cutting calories," says Keith Thomas Ayoob, a nutritionist at the Albert Einstein College of Medicine in New York. Proof of this assertion comes from a study conducted by researchers in the Department of Nutritional Sciences at the University of Oklahoma. They divided a group of people into three diets: an Atkins-like low-carbohydrate, high-protein diet; the Zone diet; and a conventional diet that restricted calories. The program lasted 3 months, and those participating had an average weight loss of 11 pounds no matter what diet they were on. At the end of the study, "there were no significant differences in total weight, fat, or lean body mass when compared by diet group," say the researchers. It was calorie control that made the difference in weight loss.

In another study conducted by researchers at Stanford University and Yale University, and published in 2003 in the *Journal of the American Medical Association*, scientists reviewed 107 studies on diets involving more than 3000 people. They found that people who lose weight on low-carb diets do so because of "reduced calories, not carbohydrate restriction." ✗ ⅄

Fortunately, the Calcium Key Weight-Loss Plan is not a fad. It's based on scientific facts. When we put groups of people on calorie-restricted diets with and without dairy foods, we found that those on the dairy diet lost 70% more weight than those who just restricted calories.

Cutting Calories the Easy Way

You need to be conscious of calories, but you don't need to deprive yourself with a low-calorie diet that cuts out all your favorite foods. The Calcium Key Weight-Loss Plan will show you how to easily and quickly calculate your personal maintenance level of calories—how many calories a day you need to maintain your weight. Once you've figured that out, you can choose the Calcium Key Week-by-Week Meal Plan that lets you reduce calories very slightly—about 500 calories a day below your maintenance level. That's the level of calorie restriction we used at the University of Tennessee in testing the Calcium Key Weight-Loss Plan—a level that helped a lot of people lose a whole lot of weight and body fat. And, if you want to speed up your rate of weight loss, the plan offers a "Quick Start" level of calorie restriction.

Will those 500 calories be hard to cut? Probably not as hard as you think. The recipes in *The Calcium Key* contain the levels of carbohydrates, fats, and proteins that most North Americans are already eating: 49% carbs, 35% fat, 16% protein. The diet in *The Calcium Key* isn't low-fat or low-carbohydrate or high-protein. It's normal. Which means you probably won't have to change your eating style.

Additionally, the plan uses the Calcium Key Exchange System (explained later in this chapter), which is a simple way to control calories without having to count them. All we're asking is for you to be aware of calories as you go through your first few weeks of the plan. Then you'll be pounds lighter, with less fat on your body (particularly around your middle), and you'll understand that it's easy to be conscious of calories, particularly when your fat cells are burning them 70% faster than before!

Ensure Lasting Weight Loss

Lose it fast and gain it back—that's the repetitious and self-defeating cycle of most diets. Gradual weight loss achieves permanent success. We don't mean at a snail's pace. When you go on the Calcium Key Weight-Loss Plan, it's likely you'll lose 1 to 1½ pounds a week, or 4 to 6 pounds in the first month, and every month thereafter until you're at your ideal weight. Those who choose the Quick-Start Plan can expect to lose 8 to 10 pounds in the first month. No matter which level of the plan you choose, you'll not only lose those pounds, you'll keep them off.

How Not to Lose Lots of Water and Muscle

When you try to lose weight as quickly as possible by cutting calories drastically (and that's the only way to force rapid weight loss, no matter what some diet books claim), your body doesn't know you're on a diet. All your body knows is that it's no longer getting the energy—the fuel, the calories—that it needs to function.

Your body is an evolutionary creature—a self-preservation mechanism designed for survival. If it can't get fuel from food, it gets fuel from someplace else, even if it has to use itself for fuel, which is exactly what happens when you try to achieve too-rapid weight loss with too-few calories.

First, your body burns stored carbohydrates. (Burning carbohydrates also gets rid of some of the water that is bound with those carbs. That's why you may lose a lot of water weight in the first few days of any very low-calorie diet.) But there's only a limited supply of stored carbs.

Next, your body burns fat. In evolutionary terms, fat is used for nutritional emergencies—survival during a famine, for example—which means your body always burns fat at a slow, survive-as-long-as-possible rate that you can't speed up no matter how few calories you eat. Because stored fat burns slowly, your underfed body has to turn to other sources of fuel to meet its immediate needs. Your vital organs are out of bounds, of course—burning up heart muscle won't help keep you alive. But losing a little skeletal muscle—the muscles attached to the bones, the muscles that help your body move—won't kill you. So, that's what your body burns next.

Losing skeletal muscle may not be deadly, but in terms of maintaining weight loss, it's self-defeating. Under normal circumstances, your skeletal muscles aren't used for calories; they burn calories. Lots of calories. Lose weight too fast, lose calorie-incinerating skeletal muscle, and when you resume eating a normal level of calories, you'll see your weight quickly return. That's the self-defeating process experienced by millions of dieters who lose weight too fast—an experience they have again . . . and again . . . and again.

- If you lose weight too fast, you lose mostly water and skeletal muscle. That's bad for you.
- If you lose weight gradually, you lose fat. That's good for you.

The Calcium Key Weight-Loss Plan helps you lose weight gradually, ensuring the pounds you lose are the pounds you want to lose: pounds of fat.

Too-Fast Weight Loss Increases Appetite and Decreases Calorie Burning

The body has other ways of responding to a drastic reduction of calories that don't help you lose weight. When you try to lose weight too fast, your body manufactures less *leptin,* a hormone that regulates appetite and metabolism, the rate at which you burn calories. Leptin is another evolutionary device to help protect the body during periods when it doesn't get enough food. It decreases appetite and increases metabolism. When calorie levels are way too low, lower levels of leptin cause you to eat a lot more food and burn fewer calories. That's exactly the opposite of what you want to happen when you're trying to lose weight! Weight-loss programs that succeed satisfy your appetite and increase the rate at which you burn calories.

Gain Health Fast with Gradual Weight Loss

Another reason for gradual weight loss is that losing a lot of weight really fast isn't necessary to quickly accomplish your health goals. Research shows that losing only 5 to 10% of your total weight dramatically lowers your risk for a number of diseases, including heart disease, stroke, high blood pressure, diabetes, and other chronic health problems. For example, a 200-pound woman who is 80 pounds overweight needs to lose only 10 pounds to reduce her risk of dying from a chronic disease by 20%.

In a study conducted at the Baylor College of Medicine in Houston and published in *Diabetes and Obesity Metabolism,* researchers looked at the effect of a small degree of weight loss on overweight people with the various health problems that constitute metabolic syndrome: high blood pressure; high levels of glucose, or blood sugar (a risk factor for diabetes); high levels of triglycerides (a blood fat); low levels of HDL, or good cholesterol; and excessive amounts of abdominal fat. Having metabolic syndrome is itself a risk factor for developing heart disease and type II (adult-onset) diabetes.

The people in the study lost only 6.5% of their weight, but their blood pressure decreased, their glucose levels fell, and their blood fats normalized. "Moderate weight loss," say the researchers, "improved all aspects of the metabolic syndrome."

Researchers at the University of Glasgow in Scotland studied 29 overweight people with angina—the chest pain that is a symptom of heart disease and a possible warning sign of an impending heart attack. An average weight loss of only 4% cut the frequency of angina attacks from 3.2 episodes per week to 1.4.

In a study conducted by Italian researchers and published in the *European Journal of Clinical Nutrition,* 268 people who lost just 4% of their weight experienced an array of health benefits: lower total cholesterol, higher HDL cholesterol, and lower blood pressure.

Lose Weight Gradually and Keep It Off for Good

Scientific studies of dieters show that the more gradually they reduce weight, the more likely they are to keep it off. In a study conducted at Rutgers University and published in the *International Journal of Obesity and Related Metabolic Disorders,* the researchers evaluated the success of the Trevose behavior modification program, which emphasizes some of the same lifestyle changes as the Calcium Key Weight-Loss Plan: awareness of calories, regular exercise, and gradual weight loss. The study showed that those who stuck with the program for 2 years lost an average of 19% of their body weight; at 5 years, the average loss was 17%.

A major reason that this type of gradual weight loss works is that you have time to learn and make a new habit of healthier ways of eating and exercising that guarantee you years rather than months of weight-loss success. A lifestyle, not a diet, allows you to maintain weight loss.

Phyllis's Story: The Only Diet That Ever Worked

Phyllis, a 36-year-old mother of three and owner of a day care center, was a participant in one of our weight-loss studies at the University of Tennessee. She started the Calcium Key Weight-Loss Plan at 180 pounds and is down to 159 pounds. And she has lost 5 inches from her waistline. She had tried lots of diets, from Fat Flush to Atkins, and this is the only weight-loss plan she has ever been on that has really worked.

One of the features Phyllis liked the most about the Calcium Key Weight-Loss Plan was keeping a food diary. By writing down everything she ate, she found it easy to stay on the plan. She also liked the free food—the no-limit low-cal foods in the Calcium Key Exchange System. She would put some cucumbers and low-fat salad dressing in a plastic container and take that with her to work, munching on the veggies whenever she felt hungry.

Getting three servings a day of dairy was no problem for Phyllis. She had a piece of cheese a day as a snack in the morning or afternoon. She would have milk with her cereal every morning. And she had yogurt every day, usually with lunch and sometimes as a midafternoon snack.

"This is a great diet," she told me. "It gave me everything it promised, and I can't say that about any of the other diets I've tried."

Tame Your Appetite with High-Volume Foods

It seems like it would be easy to satisfy your appetite. To feel full at the end of a meal. To feel like you aren't hungry anymore. To stop eating because you want to stop. To have the experience that scientists who study hunger and appetite call satiety.

Unfortunately, for most of us, satiety is not on the menu. Sure, you can feel good while eating. And stuffed if you eat too much. But feeling really satisfied after an ordinary meal probably happens once or twice a week at most.

And so, if you're like many North Americans, you eat more in order to feel satisfied. You eat big portions; you snack between meals. That means that day after day your calorie equation doesn't add up—you take in a lot more calories than you burn. And, in spite of what some diet docs tell you, those calories count. As you read earlier, research shows that the metabolic boost of the Calcium Key Weight-Loss Plan will work only if you don't overdo it on calories.

Scientists have found that it's not any particular food or any ingredient in food that creates satiety. It's mainly the volume of food you eat. If you eat the following foods, which are high in volume and relatively low in calories, you may find yourself eating a lot more food, feeling full after meals and not having as much trouble controlling your weight:

- Whole grains, like rice, oats, and wheat (cooked grains, breads, pasta, and high-fiber breakfast cereals)
- Vegetables and fruits (with the exception of dried fruits, which are high in calories)
- Legumes (dry beans, peas, chickpeas, lentils, and soy foods)
- Lean fish (like tuna and halibut) and seafood (like shrimp)
- Lean poultry (turkey is leaner than chicken) and veal
- Egg substitutes and eggs (not fried)

The amount or volume of food is the key principle in satisfying appetite. But some satiety studies also show that protein may produce the most satiety among the macronutrients (proteins, fats, and carbohydrates). Whey, a protein in milk, may be particularly satisfying.

Many studies using milk have been conducted by appetite scientists at Pennsylvania State University, led by Barbara Rolls, Ph.D., professor of nutrition, past president of the North American Association for the Study of Obesity, a leading researcher on the link between high-volume, low-calorie foods and appetite and weight loss, and author of *Volumetrics: Feel Full on Fewer Calories.* Rolls's work shows that drinking milk before or with a meal helps you feel full sooner at that meal and eat less at the next meal.

Kenneth Koch, M.D., a gastroenterologist and professor of medicine at Pennsylvania State College of Medicine, explains milk's satiety-producing ability this way: "Milk turns to a semisolid in the stomach, which means there's more neuromuscular work that must be done. This increases the satiety signals going to the brain that say you're not on empty anymore. When you drink a glass of milk, you're not hungry for a while."

And it's not just full-fat milk that does the trick. Rolls's research shows that fat-free skim milk works better than low-fat (1% fat) milk, which works better than reduced-fat (2% fat) milk. That's because diluting the calories—when full-fat milk becomes reduced, low-, or nonfat milk—increases the volume of the drink and therefore its appetite-satisfying effect.

Rolls's advice for using milk to help achieve satiety is to drink an 8-ounce glass of skim milk before a meal. She also recommends a between-meal snack of a smoothie made with nonfat yogurt, crushed ice, strawberries, and a banana. Smoothies are so effective in delivering a delicious serving of dairy and in helping you feel full that I've included 10 recipes for dairy-rich smoothies in this book.

Start with Soup

Soup creates satiety in just about every way a food can, explains Rolls. Your eyes see a big portion that you expect to be filling. It has a steamy aroma. (Studies show that the more a food looks, tastes, and smells good—in other words, the more it involves your senses—the more satisfying it is.) The soup's large volume fills up your stomach, sending messages to the brain that you're full. If the soup contains high-fiber whole grains, vegetables, legumes, or low-fat milk, it will leave your stomach slowly, triggering hormones that tell your brain you're not hungry.

Another reason that soup is so good at satisfying your appetite is its high water content. In a study published in the *American Journal of Clinical Nutrition,* Rolls and her colleagues at Penn State fed 24 women lunch in their laboratory 1 day a week for 4 weeks. Before each lunch, the women received one of three 270-calorie dishes: a chicken rice casserole; the casserole plus a 10-ounce glass of water; or a chicken rice soup made with exactly the same ingredients as the casserole served with water. Of the three dishes, the soup produced the most satiety, reducing by an average of 100 calories the amount of food the women ate at lunch. And the women who ate the soup didn't eat extra food at dinner to make up for the missing calories.

Perhaps the best type of soup to help you feel satisfied is one with lots of chunky, chewy ingredients. In a study by French researchers published in the journal *Appetite,* a group of 22 men ate a dish of either vegetables and water, strained vegetable soup, or chunky vegetable soup. All three meals were identical in calories and ingredients, and all three reduced hunger and the amount of food the men ate at the next meal. But the chunky soup reduced hunger and food intake the most.

There are many appetite-taming soups you can eat as a first course or snack, like minestrone, potato leek, corn chowder, mushroom barley, roast turkey, or gazpacho. You can also try milk-containing soups such as cream of broccoli, cream of mushroom, or tomato soup (use low-fat or fat-free milk and just a dollop of sour cream).

Fill Up on Fiber

Foods high in fiber, particularly whole grains, vegetables, fruits, and legumes, are among your best allies in taming appetite. High-fiber foods give you a lot of volume for very few calories. They fill you up, and that sensation of fullness can last for 8 to 12 hours after a meal.

Fiber-rich whole grains should be a significant part of your diet. In Rolls's analysis of the energy density (the amount of calories per gram of food) of bread and grain products, it was Spanish rice, wild rice, and long-grain brown rice that had the three lowest levels of energy density. "Rice has been a staple in cultures that have been thin for millennia," she says.

A high-fiber breakfast is one of the easiest and best ways to get your fiber. In *Volumetrics,* Rolls cites a study in which people who ate a high-fiber breakfast also ate fewer calories at breakfast and at lunch, totaling about 150 less calories for the day. Other research shows that those who eat breakfast rather than skipping it are more successful at losing weight.

Grains are an excellent source of fiber. Fruits and vegetables, of course, are also loaded with fiber and are low in calories.

There's even more good news about fiber and weight loss. In a study published in the *Journal of the American Medical Association,* researchers analyzed the daily diet and patterns of weight gain in 3000 people who had participated in a 10-year study on risk factors of heart disease. They found that dietary fiber had a very strong protective effect against weight gain. In fact, they found that the amount of fiber that people ate was a more important factor in determining who did or didn't gain weight than the amount of fat they ate.

Don't Skimp on Protein

Calorie for calorie, protein may provide more satiety than carbohydrates or fat, says Anthony Tremblay, Ph.D., chief of the Kinesiology Division at Laval University in Quebec, Canada. In a study published in the *European Journal of Clinical Nutrition,* Tremblay and his colleagues gave overweight men either high-protein (30% calories from protein) or moderate-protein (15% calories from protein) meals for 6 days, allowing them to eat as much as they liked. The men eating the high-protein meals had the most satiety, consumed the fewest calories, and lost the most weight.

Among red meat, poultry, and fish, it's possible that fish may produce the most satiety, says Rolls. She cites a study published in the *Journal of Nutrition* in which men were fed protein meals derived from beef, chicken, or fish—in the 3 hours after the meal, fish produced the greatest sense of fullness. In Rolls's analysis of the energy density of meat, poultry, and fish, tuna canned in water scores just about the lowest, delivering the fewest calories for size of almost any of these protein foods. For example, tuna has an energy density of 1.1, while bacon has an energy density of 5.0.

Hot Peppers Are Surprisingly Satisfying

While I don't think that red pepper is anywhere near as effective in controlling appetite as high-volume, low-calorie foods, research does show that it can spice up your satiety strategy. In a series of experiments published in the *British Journal of Nutrition,* Tremblay and his colleagues added red pepper to either breakfast or appetizers at a lunch and measured how much people ate afterward. He also measured how many additional calories they burned and how much additional fat they burned.

In testing 13 women, he found the addition of red pepper to a breakfast significantly reduced hunger after breakfast and before lunch and significantly decreased the consumption of calories at lunch. When he tested 10 men, he found the addition of red pepper to an appetizer eaten before lunch significantly reduced calorie intake during lunch and in a snack that was served a few hours later.

Tremblay says the red pepper acts as a nonpharmacological stimulant (there's a long history of using stimulating drugs like caffeine to control appetite), boosting the activity of the sympathetic nervous system so that you feel less hungry. As an added bonus, Tremblay found that red pepper significantly increased both calories and fat burned, particularly after a high-fat meal. And red pepper improved the perceived oiliness of a low-fat meal so that it seemed more like a high-fat meal. "Red pepper might provide low-fat foods with a texture that makes them very similar to high-fat foods," he says.

Combining spicy salsa with vegetables is a particularly good way to get your hot peppers, since vegetables (along with fruit) have a water content of 80 to 95%, plus lots of fiber, putting them at the center of any high-volume, low-calorie eating plan.

Use the Glycemic Index to Stop Stuffing Your Fat Cells

Now you're going to learn the straightforward scientific facts about carbohydrates—those sugars and starches that some diet doctors say are the #1 cause of overweight. The most important fact: not all carbs are the same.

Yes, all sugars and starches—whether we're talking about the sugar in honey or the starch in potatoes—break down in the small intestine to form the simplest carbohydrate: glucose, or blood sugar. Glucose is the main fuel for the cells in the body.

Some foods high in carbohydrates, like instant rice, break down quickly during digestion. That's bad for weight control. Some foods high in carbohydrates, like brown rice, break down slowly during digestion. That's good for weight control.

Why would the rate at which a food turns into glucose determine whether it's your waistline's friend or enemy? A dish that contains mostly quick-digesting carbs, like the refined grain of white bread or the sugar in soda, can generate twice as much blood sugar as a meal containing mostly slow-digesting carbs, like fruits, vegetables, beans, and whole grains. When that happens, the pancreas manufactures extra insulin, the hormone that escorts blood sugar out of the bloodstream and into the cells. The extra dose of insulin pushes extra amounts of blood sugar into fat cells. A lot of that sugar is turned into fat. Extra sugar also inhibits the ability of fat cells to burn fat. If you eat enough meals with enough fast-digesting carbs, your fat cells will make more fat and burn less. Not surprisingly, you're likely to get fatter.

How Quickly Foods Turn into Glucose

In the early 1980s, a Canadian scientist and expert on fiber, David Jenkins, M.D., Ph.D., invented an index to quantify how slowly or quickly the carbohydrates in foods turn into glucose. It's called the glycemic index (GI). The top number on the index is 100, the rate at which food turns into glucose. Almost every other number on the index is less than 100: higher numbers for foods that turn into glucose quickly; lower numbers for foods that turn into glucose slowly. For example,

- Kellogg's All-Bran has a GI value of 30; Kellogg's Cocoa Puffs, 77.
- Brown rice has a GI value of 50; instant rice, 87.
- Baked beans have a GI value of 48; jelly beans, 78.
- Milk has a GI value of 27; ice cream, 61.
- Peanuts have a GI value of 14; potato chips, 57.

High-GI foods trigger your body to produce and store more fat. Low-GI foods are much less likely to do that. Also, low-GI foods satisfy your appetite and delay hunger. The Calcium Key Weight-Loss Plan encourages you to maximize low-GI foods and minimize high-GI foods.

In an article in the *Journal of Nutrition* summarizing research on overweight and the GI, David S. Ludwig, M.D., a Harvard-based researcher, says, "Diets designed to lower the insulin response to ingested carbohydrate (low GI) may . . . decrease hunger, and promote weight loss." A diet that emphasizes low-GI foods can help you stay slim. But it may also help you stay alive. Studies show that low-GI diets are linked to a decreased risk of developing diabetes and heart disease.

Dairy Foods: Very Low on the Glycemic Index

Almost all dairy foods are low-GI foods. When you eat a dairy food, a protein curd forms in the stomach, slowing down the rate at which the food is digested. Dairy foods have carbohydrates, fats, and proteins. Fats and proteins slow digestion, further lowering the GI of dairy foods. Milk has a GI of 31. Yogurt has a GI of 14 to 36, depending on the brand (artificially sweetened brands have lower GI values).

Dairy foods are not only an important low-GI part of every meal but a perfect substitute for high-GI midmorning and midafternoon snacks like sodas and candy bars. In the long run, those types of snacks can make you hungrier and fatter. But a small piece of cheese, a cup of low-fat yogurt, or a glass of reduced-fat chocolate milk are satisfying when you eat them and you'll feel satisfied longer.

Simple Guidelines for a Low-GI Diet

Putting the GI into practice is easy. You don't have to be concerned about meals that mix low-GI and high-GI foods. If you emphasize low-GI foods in your diet, you shouldn't worry about the high-GI foods you also include. Here are the basics of a low-GI diet, as found in the meal plans and recipes of the Calcium Key Weight-Loss Plan:

- Increase your intake of dairy foods (low GI).
- Increase your intake of fruits and vegetables (low GI).
- Increase your intake of beans and peas (low GI).
- Choose grain products that are whole (low or medium GI) rather than refined (high GI). Choose whole-wheat bread over white bread, steel-cut or rolled oats (two forms of whole oats) over precooked instant, and brown rice over white. Include lots of whole grains in your diet, like buckwheat, millet, and barley (low GI).
- Limit your intake of potatoes (high GI).
- Limit your intake of concentrated sugar, like that found in soda, candy, doughnuts, and other sweetened baked goods (high GI).

Don't Believe the Myths about Low-Fat Food

Let's look at the fat content of different varieties of milk:

- Fat-free (0%) or skim milk has 5% of its calories from fat.
- Low-fat (1%) or light milk has 18% of its calories from fat.
- Reduced-fat milk (2%) has 34% of its calories from fat.
- Whole milk (3.5%) has 48% of its calories from fat.

The Calcium Key Weight-Loss Plan recommends you consume mostly no-, low-, and reduced-fat dairy foods. Overall, the plan isn't low in fat. It delivers 49% of its calories from carbohydrates, 16% from protein, and 35% from fat.

If the entire plan isn't low in fat, why recommend low-fat dairy foods? Because having 3 to 4 servings a day of full-fat dairy could make it difficult for you to decrease your total calories. As you know, it's too many calories, not too much fat, that is the problem with the North American diet.

Case in point. The fat content of the North American diet has been dropping. But the fat content of North American bodies has been rising.

A low-fat diet has been proposed as a simple solution to the complex problem of overweight and ill health. But fat in food was never a villain in your daily diet. Although huge quantities of fat are bad, fat can be a hero if you eat the right amounts and right kinds.

"The Soft Science of Dietary Fat," an award-winning article by journalist Gary Taubes, published in *Science,* points out that the scientific facts underlying the recommendations for a low-fat diet are quite weak, maybe even nonexistent. For example, in 1988, the U.S. Surgeon General's Office tried to write a report on the evils of dietary fat. Over a decade later, the

project was killed for lack of definitive evidence supporting the precon-
ceived conclusion that fat is bad for you.

Fat Content Down, Heart Problems Up

Many public health officials and organizations recommend a low-fat diet
because they believe that decreasing overall fat, particularly the saturated fat
found in meat and dairy foods, protects you against heart disease. But does
it? A survey from the U.S. Department of Agriculture shows that since the
early 1970s the calories from fat in the average American diet have dropped
from 40% to 33%, and the saturated fat content from 18% to 11%. During
this same period, the number of medical procedures for heart disease has
increased from 1.2 million to 5.4 million a year. Some recent scientific studies show that total fat intake may have no relation to heart disease. Other
studies indicate that monounsaturated fats (found in olive oil, for example)
help protect your heart, while trans fats (found in baked goods and margarine) may be more harmful than saturated fat.

Low-Fat Is Not the Answer to Weight Loss

Fifty thousand women in the government's Women's Health Initiative program were counseled to eat a very low-fat diet—20% of calories from fat.
After 3 years, the women had lost an average of 2.2 pounds. This is only one
of many studies showing that low-fat diets don't necessarily work.

Researchers at the Harvard School of Public Health and the Columbia
University College of Physicians and Surgeons looked at several scientifically rigorous long-term studies on low-fat diets and weight loss. Writing in
the *American Journal of Medicine,* the researchers say the studies show low-
fat diets don't work. The bottom line: whether dieters ate as few as 18% of
calories from fat or as much as 40%, the diets had "little if any effect on
body fatness." They conclude: "Within the United States, a substantial
decline in the percentage of energy from fat during the last 2 decades has
corresponded with a massive increase in obesity. Diets high in fat do not
appear to be the primary cause of the high prevalence of excess body fat in
our society, and reductions in fat will not be a solution."

The Risk of Too Many Carbohydrates

That a low-fat diet doesn't lead to better health and weight loss is only part
of the problem. It may actually cause weight gain.

Low-fat diets are usually high-carbohydrate diets. Too often, those
carbohydrates are what nutritionists call *simple*—sugary, low-fiber, high-
calorie foods (like low-fat cookies) that don't fill you up. Your body has an

efficient mechanism for turning excess calories, including calories from car-bohydrates, into body fat. So, if you overeat low-fat, high-calorie foods, you're going to gain weight. That's what North Americans have been doing.

Go Ahead—Eat the Percentage of Calories from Fat That You're Already Eating

Scientific evidence says that a low-fat, high-calorie diet is not the answer to weight loss or good health. It says that a low-fat diet can actually promote weight gain and can cause health problems if simple carbohydrates are sub-stituted for fat.

You're likely to discover that the amazing change in your fat cells as you eat 3 to 4 daily servings of calcium-rich dairy foods creates and sustains suc-cessful weight loss. Your cells will lower their fat production, making less fat, storing less fat, and burning more fat. You'll lower fat levels where it really counts—in your body, not in your diet.

3

Calcium Key Weight-Loss Success

IN THIS CHAPTER, you'll learn the meal-by-meal and day-by-day details of the Calcium Key Weight-Loss Plan: what it is and how to do it.

First, I'll introduce you to the calorie levels of the plan—a level for every lifestyle and desired speed of weight loss. You'll go through a simple three-step process to find out which level is right for you.

Next, I'll explain the Calcium Key Exchange System (CKES) and show you how to use it. CKES is the practical essence of the plan.

After CKES, you'll find the High-Dairy Calcium Guide, which provides you with an extensive list of dairy foods, along with their calcium, fat, and calorie contents. This list will help inform and expand your choices as you get your 3 to 4 servings of dairy a day.

The chapter closes with a discussion about an important topic: how people who are lactose intolerant—who sometimes get mild digestive upset when they consume dairy—can follow the Calcium Key Weight-Loss Plan with virtually no symptoms or discomfort.

Figure Out Your Weight-Loss Calorie Level and Get Started

The three-step process of figuring out your weight-loss calorie level is very easy because this section provides extensive tables with daily maintenance calorie levels for women and men of every weight, age, and degree of physical activity. These tables will allow you to easily do step 1—figure out how many calories a day you need to maintain your weight—and therefore move easily to steps 2 and 3. Before you can use the tables, however, you need a little more information about the different ways in which your body burns calories.

The Three Ways Your Body Burns Calories

The first and most significant way is your *resting metabolic rate (RMR)*—the level of calories you burn to maintain your everyday bodily functions, like breathing, heartbeat, blood circulation, and temperature. RMR accounts for the calories you burn when you're not doing much of anything, like when you're asleep. It comprises 60 to 70% of the calories you burn.

A man has a higher RMR than a woman, and RMR decreases with age. The tables for determining maintenance calories are based in part on RMR and therefore take into account the differences between men and women, and between age groups.

You also burn calories by the *thermic effects of foods (TEF)*—the level of calories you burn as your body digests and otherwise processes food. This accounts for about 5 to 10% of the calories you burn in a day.

TEF changes with the type of food you eat. You burn more calories when you digest carbohydrates or protein than you do when you digest fat. Spicy foods can increase TEF; so can caffeine.

However, getting an accurate count of your TEF, which varies from meal to meal, requires daily food records and complex computations. For simplicity's sake, I used an average TEF to devise the maintenance calorie information.

Another way you burn calories is *physical activity.* Somebody who is confined to bed burns about 10% of his or her daily calories from physical activity. An elite athlete in training burns as much as 50% of daily calories from physical activity.

Your Level of Physical Activity

For the purpose of figuring out your maintenance calories, you'll need to decide which level of physical activity describes you best:

1. Low activity
2. Moderate activity
3. Strenuous activity

Low activity means you have a job where you sit or stand most of the day—you're an office worker, for example, rather than a construction worker. Besides being sedentary at work, you're sedentary before and after work, meaning you don't exercise regularly.

Moderate activity means you have a sedentary job, but you exercise a couple of days a week. You do 45 or more minutes of an aerobic activity that gets your heart beating faster, like brisk walking, jogging, bicycling, or swimming. Moderate activity can also mean that you have an active rather than a sedentary job but don't exercise.

Strenuous activity means you exercise at least 5 days a week.

If you overestimate your activity level, your estimate of your maintenance level of calories will be too high. You'll pick a CKES that is too high in calories to help you shed pounds. Studies show that many people overestimate their level of physical activity when asked for an estimate, so please be realistic. For example, an office job where you walk to the copy machine a couple of times a day is not an active job. An active job is one where the job itself is active. Postal clerks have a sedentary job; postal carriers have an active job.

Likewise, be realistic about your level of exercise. Don't base your estimate on what you plan to do next week. Base it on what you've done consistently over the past couple of months.

Using the Tables

Now that you know how to estimate your level of physical activity, you'll need to figure out your maintenance level of calories. Let's say you're a 42-year-old woman who weighs 162 pounds. You have a job where you sit all day, and you exercise three times a week for 30 minutes. Your activity level is moderate.

Go to the table for women 31 to 60 years old and find the weight that is closest to 162 pounds. Average up or down to the closest number. For this example, at 162 pounds you'd use the 160-pound weight. If you weighed 163 pounds, you'd use the 165-pound weight.

Now, move from the weight at the left of the table to the right, finding the number in the moderate activity column at 160 pounds. That number is: 2135 calories.

1. Use your own age, weight, and level of physical activity, and figure out your maintenance level of calories.
2. Subtract 500 calories from your maintenance level of calories. In the example, that number would be 1635 calories. Calculate your own number.
3. Choose the Calcium Key Exchange System that is closest to the number derived from step 2. In the example, it would be the 1600-calorie CKES.

If you choose the Quick-Start Calcium Key Plan, you could have one more step. Let's look at that option.

The Quick-Start Calcium Key Plan

In conducting studies at the University of Tennessee, we helped lots of people lose lots of weight by cutting their daily calorie intake to a level 500 calories below their maintenance level and adding 3 servings of dairy a day to the diet.

If you cut calories by 500 a day and eat 3 servings of dairy a day, you'll lose about 1 to 1½ pounds a week, or 4 to 6 pounds in the first month. However, you may want to see quicker results.

If that's the case, choose the Quick-Start Plan by cutting your calorie intake to 1000 calories below your maintenance level. If you choose this plan, you'll lose about 2 to 2½ pounds per week, or 8 to 10 pounds in the first month.

In the example we just used, you would subtract 1000 calories from 2135, putting you at 1135. In that case, you would choose the 1200-calorie Calcium Key Exchange System.

Don't go below the 1200-calorie Calcium Key Exchange System. The calorie level is too low for you to be optimally healthy.

As I said earlier, drastically restricting calories burns up more skeletal muscle than fat. Losing skeletal muscle interferes with long-term weight loss. That's because the activity of skeletal muscle uses up a lot of calories under normal circumstances.

Also, restricting calories below 1200 a day is very restrictive. It's likely that such a dramatic decrease in food intake will leave you feeling deprived. And deprivation leads to its opposite: overdoing it. An extremely restricted diet is usually followed by an extremely unrestricted diet.

I want you to lose weight permanently. I want you to free yourself from the self-defeating, frustrating cycle so common among dieters: diet, binge, diet, binge; lose, gain, lose, gain. To lose weight permanently, it's best to lose weight gradually, which is most easily accomplished by cutting 500 calories from your maintenance level.

But whether you subtract 500 or 1000 calories from your maintenance level, you're going to be adding 3 servings of dairy a day to your diet. And that is going to make a huge difference in your body's ability to burn fat and your ability to lose weight.

Noel's Story: Cheese, Tea, and Weight Loss

Noel had no problem getting his dairy on the Calcium Key Weight-Loss Plan. Noel loved tea. The 42-year-old appliance salesman drank eight or nine cups of tea a day, always with milk. That provided him with about 8 ounces of milk, or 1 dairy exchange. He switched to skim, which he found a little bit trying until he got used to it. He also loved sharp white cheddar cheese, so he'd have two slices of that a day. Every now and then, he'd cheat and have an extra slice or two, and go a little bit over his fat exchanges. But that didn't stop Noel from losing weight.

He was really determined to lose his extra pounds, he told me. And he found it easy, because all he had to do was count his exchanges. He loved a glass of whisky in the evening, which counted as 1½ bread exchanges.

The result of following the Calcium Key Exchange System was that Noel lost over 30 pounds. He started at 211 and is now at 179. And he has lost 4 inches off his belly.

Noel asked me to pass on these words of encouragement: "Doc, tell them they can lose weight if they stick with the Calcium Key Weight-Loss Plan. It works. It really does."

FIGURE OUT YOUR MAINTENANCE CALORIE LEVEL

Women 18 to 30 Years Old					Men 18 to 30 Years Old				
Weight	RMR	Low Activity	Moderate Activity	Strenuous Activity	Weight	RMR	Low Activity	Moderate Activity	Strenuous Activity
100	1231	1600	1723	1847	100	1444	1877	2022	2166
105	1268	1648	1775	1902	105	1482	1927	2075	2223
110	1305	1696	1826	1957	110	1521	1977	2129	2281
115	1341	1744	1878	2012	115	1559	2026	2182	2338
120	1378	1791	1929	2067	120	1597	2076	2236	2396
125	1415	1839	1981	2122	125	1635	2126	2289	2453
130	1452	1887	2032	2177	130	1674	2176	2343	2510
135	1488	1935	2084	2232	135	1712	2225	2397	2568
140	1525	1983	2135	2288	140	1750	2275	2450	2625
145	1562	2030	2186	2343	145	1788	2325	2504	2682
150	1599	2078	2238	2398	150	1827	2374	2557	2740
155	1635	2126	2289	2453	155	1865	2424	2611	2797
160	1672	2174	2341	2508	160	1903	2474	2664	2855
165	1709	2221	2392	2563	165	1941	2524	2718	2912
170	1746	2269	2444	2618	170	1980	2573	2771	2969
175	1782	2317	2495	2673	175	2018	2623	2825	3027
180	1819	2365	2547	2729	180	2056	2673	2878	3084
185	1856	2412	2598	2784	185	2094	2723	2932	3141
190	1893	2460	2650	2839	190	2133	2772	2986	3199
195	1929	2508	2701	2894	195	2171	2822	3039	3256
200	1966	2556	2752	2949	200	2209	2872	3093	3314
205	2003	2604	2804	3004	205	2247	2921	3146	3371
210	2040	2651	2855	3059	210	2286	2971	3200	3428
215	2076	2699	2907	3114	215	2324	3021	3253	3486
220	2113	2747	2958	3170	220	2362	3071	3307	3543
225	2150	2795	3010	3225	225	2400	3120	3360	3600
230	2187	2842	3061	3280	230	2439	3170	3414	3658
235	2223	2890	3113	3335	235	2477	3220	3468	3715
240	2260	2938	3164	3390	240	2515	3270	3521	3773
245	2297	2986	3215	3445	245	2553	3319	3575	3830
250	2334	3034	3267	3500	250	2592	3369	3628	3887

FIGURE OUT YOUR MAINTENANCE CALORIE LEVEL *(continued)*

Women 31 to 60 Years Old | Men 31 to 60 Years Old

Weight	RMR	Low Activity	Moderate Activity	Strenuous Activity	Weight	RMR	Low Activity	Moderate Activity	Strenuous Activity
100	1264	1643	1770	1896	100	1459	1897	2043	2189
105	1286	1671	1800	1929	105	1488	1934	2083	2232
110	1308	1700	1831	1961	110	1517	1972	2124	2276
115	1329	1728	1861	1994	115	1546	2010	2164	2319
120	1351	1756	1891	2027	120	1575	2048	2205	2363
125	1373	1785	1922	2059	125	1604	2085	2246	2406
130	1395	1813	1952	2092	130	1633	2123	2286	2450
135	1416	1841	1983	2124	135	1662	2161	2327	2493
140	1438	1869	2013	2157	140	1691	2198	2367	2537
145	1460	1898	2044	2190	145	1720	2236	2408	2580
150	1482	1926	2074	2222	150	1749	2274	2449	2624
155	1503	1954	2105	2255	155	1778	2311	2489	2667
160	1525	1983	2135	2288	160	1807	2349	2530	2711
165	1547	2011	2165	2320	165	1836	2387	2570	2754
170	1569	2039	2196	2353	170	1865	2425	2611	2798
175	1590	2067	2226	2385	175	1894	2462	2652	2841
180	1612	2096	2257	2418	180	1923	2500	2692	2885
185	1634	2124	2287	2451	185	1952	2538	2733	2928
190	1656	2152	2318	2483	190	1981	2575	2773	2972
195	1677	2180	2348	2516	195	2010	2613	2814	3015
200	1699	2209	2379	2549	200	2039	2651	2855	3059
205	1721	2237	2409	2581	205	2068	2688	2895	3102
210	1743	2265	2440	2614	210	2097	2726	2936	3146
215	1764	2294	2470	2646	215	2126	2764	2976	3189
220	1786	2322	2500	2679	220	2155	2802	3017	3233
225	1808	2350	2531	2712	225	2184	2839	3058	3276
230	1830	2378	2561	2744	230	2213	2877	3098	3320
235	1851	2407	2592	2777	235	2242	2915	3139	3363
240	1873	2435	2622	2810	240	2271	2952	3179	3407
245	1895	2463	2653	2842	245	2300	2990	3220	3450
250	1917	2491	2683	2875	250	2329	3028	3261	3494

The Calcium Key Exchange System: Losing Weight Was Never So Easy

Now I will introduce you to the practical essence of the Calcium Key Weight-Loss Plan, the meal-by-meal, day-by-day details of the eating program you'll use to shed fat: the Calcium Key Exchange System (CKES). But

Women 61 Years Old and Older | *Men 61 Years Old and Older*

Weight	RMR	Low Activity	Moderate Activity	Strenuous Activity	Weight	RMR	Low Activity	Moderate Activity	Strenuous Activity
100	1121	1457	1569	1682	100	1162	1511	1627	1743
105	1147	1491	1606	1721	105	1196	1555	1674	1794
110	1174	1526	1643	1760	110	1230	1599	1722	1845
115	1200	1560	1680	1800	115	1263	1642	1768	1895
120	1226	1594	1716	1839	120	1297	1686	1816	1946
125	1252	1628	1753	1878	125	1331	1730	1863	1997
130	1279	1662	1790	1918	130	1365	1775	1911	2048
135	1305	1696	1827	1957	135	1398	1817	1957	2097
140	1331	1730	1863	1997	140	1432	1862	2005	2148
145	1357	1764	1900	2036	145	1466	1906	2052	2199
150	1384	1799	1937	2075	150	1500	1950	2100	2250
155	1410	1833	1974	2115	155	1533	1993	2146	2300
160	1436	1867	2010	2154	160	1567	2037	2194	2351
165	1462	1901	2047	2193	165	1601	2081	2241	2402
170	1489	1935	2084	2233	170	1635	2126	2289	2453
175	1515	1969	2121	2272	175	1668	2168	2335	2502
180	1541	2003	2157	2312	180	1702	2213	2383	2553
185	1567	2037	2194	2351	185	1736	2257	2430	2604
190	1594	2072	2231	2390	190	1770	2301	2478	2655
195	1620	2106	2268	2430	195	1803	2344	2524	2705
200	1646	2140	2304	2469	200	1837	2388	2572	2756
205	1672	2174	2341	2508	205	1871	2432	2619	2807
210	1699	2208	2378	2548	210	1905	2477	2667	2858
215	1725	2242	2415	2587	215	1938	2519	2713	2907
220	1751	2276	2451	2627	220	1972	2564	2761	2958
225	1777	2310	2488	2666	225	2006	2608	2808	3009
230	1804	2345	2525	2705	230	2040	2652	2856	3060
235	1830	2379	2562	2745	235	2073	2695	2902	3110
240	1856	2413	2598	2784	240	2107	2739	2950	3161
245	1882	2447	2635	2823	245	2141	2783	2997	3212
250	1909	2481	2672	2863	250	2175	2828	3045	3263

rather than me telling you how great CKES is, I'll let a 40-year-old doctor named Patricia, whom you met in chapter 1, tell her story.

A Weight-Loss Success Story

Patricia lost nearly 40 pounds using CKES, dropping from 175 to 137 pounds, and from a size 16 to a size 8. She says,

> I've been on so many diets. But there's a big difference between the Calcium Key Plan and every other diet I've been on. The Calcium

Key Exchange System is *smart*—it's healthy, nutritionally balanced, and easy to follow.

Instead of being challenged by the complex task of keeping a daily total of calories, there's just a very simple process of counting a few exchanges—how many I've already had that day, and how many more I can have. Plus, CKES allows me so much flexibility when I eat out, which I love to do.

I would never go on another crazy, unhealthy diet again, a diet that isn't well balanced or one that severely restricts calories. The Calcium Key Exchange System is easy to follow. You can do it for a lifetime, not just a couple of weeks—and it *works*.

Dividing All Foods into Six Simple Groups

CKES is an eating plan that uses the principles of exchanges that were developed by the American Diabetes Association and the American Dietetic Association. Their dietary exchange system was designed to help people with diabetes keep blood sugar levels under control and to offer a sensible and easy-to-follow eating plan.

CKES is designed to help you control calories without having to count calories. It helps you eat a diet balanced in carbohydrates, fats, and proteins without needing a calculator and a full-time nutritional consultant. It keeps nutrition simple by dividing all foods into six groups based on their level of calories and their mix of carbohydrates, proteins, and fats.

Here are the six groups along with their abbreviations:

1. Dairy (D)
2. Breads and Grains (includes starchy vegetables; B/G)
3. Vegetables (nonstarchy; V)
4. Fruits (Fr)
5. Meats and Proteins (M/P)
6. Fats (F)

The foods in each group are given a value called an exchange because any food in that group can be exchanged for any other. Here are some examples:

- A cup of skim milk is 1 dairy exchange.
- A slice of wheat bread is 1 bread/grain exchange.
- A half cup of cooked carrots is 1 vegetable exchange.
- An orange is 1 fruit exchange.
- An ounce of sirloin steak is 1 meat/protein exchange.
- A teaspoon of oil is 1 fat exchange.

Extensive tables of foods for each of the six exchange groups are on pages 84 to 107. You'll also find five additional tables: Free Foods, Combination Foods, Sweets and Sugar, Alcoholic Beverages, and Coffee Drinks. These foods are either so low in calories that they're not assigned an exchange (the Free Foods) or they're a combination of various exchanges.

Each calorie level of the plan—1200, 1400, 1600, 1800, 2000, or 2200—is matched by a Calcium Key Exchange System for that level. You can find the CKES for each calorie level in the table that follows.

If you choose the 1600-calorie plan, for example, you will have a daily total of 3 dairy exchanges, 5 bread/grain exchanges, 5 vegetable exchanges, 4 fruit exchanges, 3 meat/protein exchanges, and 4 fat exchanges.

If you choose the 2000-calorie plan, you will have a daily total of 3 dairy exchanges, 7 bread/grain exchanges, 5 vegetable exchanges, 5 fruit exchanges, 4 meat/protein exchanges, and 6 fat exchanges.

Chapter 4 includes 5 weeks of meal plans for every calorie level of CKES. Chapter 5 has recipes for dishes that are part of those meals, with a list of exchanges for each recipe. If you use those meal plans and recipes for the first few weeks on the Calcium Key Exchange System, you won't have to think very much about exchanges—it's all planned out for you.

You'll find all the calorie levels of CKES here: 1200, 1400, 1600, 1800, 2000, and 2200. (If you're over 250 pounds, you may have completed step 3 and discovered that your Calcium Key Exchange System is over 2200 calories. If this is the case, simply combine the exchanges of two of the below plans. If your plan is 2400 calories, for example, combine the exchanges of two 1200-calorie plans.)

	Exchanges	Carb Grams	Carb Calories	Protein Grams	Protein Calories	Fat Grams	Fat Calories	Total Calories
1200 Calories								
Bread/Grain	3	45	180	9	36	6	54	270
Meat/Protein	2	0	0	14	56	10	90	146
Vegetable	3	15	60	6	24	0	0	84
Fruit	3	45	180	0	0	0	0	180
Dairy	3	36	144	24	96	15	135	375
Fat	3	0	0	0	0	15	135	135
Totals		141	564	53	212	46	414	1190
1400 Calories								
Bread/Grain	4	60	240	12	48	8	72	360
Meat/Protein	3	0	0	21	84	15	135	219
Vegetable	4	20	80	8	32	0	0	112

	Exchanges	Carb Grams	Carb Calories	Protein Grams	Protein Calories	Fat Grams	Fat Calories	Total Calories
1200 Calories (continued)								
Fruit	3	45	180	0	0	0	0	180
Dairy	3	36	144	24	96	15	135	375
Fat	3	0	0	0	0	15	135	135
Totals		161	644	65	260	53	477	1381
1600 Calories								
Bread/Grain	5	75	300	15	60	10	90	450
Meat/Protein	3	0	0	21	84	15	135	219
Vegetable	5	25	100	10	40	0	0	140
Fruit	4	60	240	0	0	0	0	240
Dairy	3	36	144	24	96	15	135	375
Fat	4	0	0	0	0	20	180	180
Totals		196	784	70	280	60	540	1604
1800 Calories								
Bread/Grain	6	90	360	18	72	12	108	540
Meat/Protein	4	0	0	28	112	20	180	292
Vegetable	4	20	80	8	32	0	0	112
Fruit	5	75	300	0	0	0	0	300
Dairy	3	36	144	24	96	15	135	375
Fat	4	0	0	0	0	20	180	180
Totals		221	884	78	312	67	603	1799
2000 Calories								
Bread/Grain	7	105	420	21	84	14	126	630
Meat/Protein	4	0	0	28	112	20	180	292
Vegetable	5	25	100	10	40	0	0	140
Fruit	5	75	300	0	0	0	0	300
Dairy	3	36	144	24	96	15	135	375
Fat	6	0	0	0	0	30	270	270
Totals		241	964	83	332	79	711	2007
2200 Calories								
Bread/Grain	8	120	480	24	96	16	144	720
Meat/Protein	5	0	0	35	140	25	225	365
Vegetable	6	30	120	12	48	0	0	168
Fruit	5	75	300	0	0	0	0	300
Dairy	3	36	144	24	96	15	135	375
Fat	6	0	0	0	0	30	270	270
Totals		261	1044	95	380	86	774	2198

Your Daily Food Budget

Perhaps the best way to think of CKES is as a daily food budget. You can spend your money on anything, but some items use up money a lot faster than other items. If you have a $100-a-day budget and you buy a $97 CD player first thing in the morning, you won't be buying a lot of other things that day.

In the same way, if you get up in the morning and eat a high-fat biscuit, you've spent 3 bread/grain and 2 fat exchanges. If, however, you eat an English muffin, you've only spent 2 bread/grain exchanges, saving yourself a bread/grain exchange and a fat exchange for later in the day.

If you drink a 12-ounce can of soda at your midmorning break, that's 3 fruit exchanges. Is that how you want to spend your fruit exchanges for the day? A soda isn't a bad food—there are no bad foods, only unbalanced diets. But you could choose to drink 6 ounces and use your other 1½ fruit exchanges for whole fruit. Or you could snack on 1 piece of fruit and still have 2 fruit exchanges left.

In fact, budgeting your exchanges throughout the day—eating smaller amounts of food many times during the day—is an excellent pattern of eating for successful weight loss. Eating breakfast, a midmorning snack, lunch, and a midafternoon snack helps you avoid overdoing your exchanges at dinner, when dieters often binge because they haven't eaten enough throughout the day. Eating small amounts throughout the day also helps regulate blood sugar, which means you're less likely to feel hungry, tired, and depressed—a metabolic and emotional setup for overeating.

"One of the best things about the Calcium Key Exchange system was that it taught me not to wait for the next meal to eat something," says Frank, a 47-year-old executive who lost 13 pounds on CKES. "Instead of getting hungry and then gorging myself at the next meal, I'd tide myself over with a piece of fruit or a low-fat granola bar."

As you adjust to CKES, you'll learn how to optimize your exchange budget. Remember, no food is excluded. It's not that you can't eat high-calorie items or desserts. But to stay within your daily exchange budget, you may have to eat smaller portions of high-calorie foods or make other adjustments during the day that allow you to eat a dessert that spends a lot of your exchanges.

In the sections that follow, you'll find lots of ideas for substituting low-calorie (lower-exchange) foods for high-calorie (higher-exchange) foods.

Picturing Portions

An exchange is often defined by its size, whether it's a teaspoon, ounce, or cup. However, you won't always have a scale or measuring spoon or cup handy when you're figuring out how much of a food equals 1 exchange. Instead, you'll have to visualize the exact amount. Here are some tips to help you:

- One and a half ounces of hard cheese (such as cheddar or Swiss) or 2 ounces of processed cheese (such as American cheese slices) is 1 dairy exchange. An ounce of cheese is about the size of your thumb, or an ice cube, or a stack of four dice.
- A meat exchange is 1 ounce of meat—about the size of a typical sausage patty. Three ounces of meat—3 meat exchanges—is about the size of a deck of cards, a bar of soap, or the palm of a woman's hand.
- Many exchanges are one-quarter, one-half, or two-thirds of a cup. To picture these sizes, one-quarter cup is one golf ball, one-half cup is two golf balls, two-thirds cup is a tennis ball, and one cup is a baseball. Or use your hand to picture a cup. A rounded handful is about one-half cup. A tightly balled fist is about 1 cup. Of course, everybody's hand is a different size. Measure 1 cup and compare it to your fist. And remember: a cup is 8 ounces, not a 32-ounce cup of soda.
- A teaspoon of butter, margarine, or oil is 1 fat exchange. A teaspoon is about the size of the tip of your thumb.
- There are 3 teaspoons in 1 tablespoon.

To help you estimate portions accurately when you're preparing a meal at home, measure out a portion—say, a cup—using a measuring cup. Then put that portion into one of the plates, bowls, or cups you use to serve food. This will help you picture if the portions you're eating are really 1 cup—or a lot more. As you follow CKES for a while, you'll find that estimating portions gets easier and easier.

Keeping a Food Diary

If you want to optimize CKES, the best strategy is to write down everything you eat. I advise you to keep a meal-by-meal, snack-by-snack food diary. When you've lost all the weight you want to lose, when you're thinner and healthier, you'll see the diary as one of your most helpful and supportive friends.

"I keep my food diary with me all the time, in my purse," says Patricia, the doctor who lost 38 pounds on CKES. "When I go out to eat, I write down what I'm eating. At home, I keep it on my kitchen counter. I consider it the single most important behavioral tool for achieving my weight-loss goals and for maintaining my weight."

In our studies at the University of Tennessee, we have found that many people in the initial stages of the study were not very detailed about recording their foods in a diary—the portions or the kinds of food. And if they weren't detailed, they usually didn't lose weight, because their estimates of their exchanges weren't accurate and therefore their calorie level was too high. They weren't actually on a plan that was 500 calories below their maintenance level. Unbeknownst to them, they were on a much higher calorie plan.

In fact, we have found that when people begin keeping a food diary, they are surprised—even amazed—by how much they are eating. Writing down what you eat makes you very aware of your exchanges. This awareness lets you actually follow your chosen Calcium Key Exchange System.

Also, as you write down what you eat during the day, you will begin to develop a food budget that makes the most sense for you. Rather than eating most of your exchanges at breakfast and lunch, you'll learn to spread them throughout the day and evening. I encourage you to subtotal your exchanges as you go through the day. This will help you stay aware of whether you're on the plan. Keeping a diary will help you see exactly when and where you exceed your exchanges, if you do.

It's crucial to write down when you eat. My colleagues and I have found that when people on CKES try to go back and remember what they ate that morning or yesterday, they can't. Write down every single thing you put in your mouth.

What was the cut of meat? Did the chicken have skin? Was the fish broiled or fried? If you ate at a fast-food restaurant, did you ask them to hold the mayonnaise?

Write down the time you ate, the amount you ate, the food item you ate, and calculate the exchanges. And don't do it at the end of the day. Total as you go.

At the end of the day, see if your total number of exchanges matches your prescribed exchange level. If it doesn't, adjust accordingly the next day.

Of course, if you use the week-by-week meal plans in this book, you won't have to adjust anything. They're tailored to give you the correct number of exchanges for your level of calorie intake.

To help you keep your food diary, I've included some useful items. There are two sample food diaries, so you can see how it's done when it's done right and, to get you started, some blank diaries of the type we give our participants in weight-loss studies at the University of Tennessee.

Sample Food Diaries

As explained, recording what you eat and drink at the time you eat and drink it is the most accurate way to keep track of your food exchanges. If you can't record your food intake at the same time you eat a meal or snack, record it as soon as possible before you forget the all-important details.

The two sample food diaries were filled out by people on the 1400-calorie CKES and the 2200-calorie CKES.

There are also blank food diaries; use them to start your diary, keeping one blank for photocopying. Or use a small lined spiral notebook and fill out a two-page spread with the same information in the sample food diaries. Put *Time, Amount,* and *Food* on the top of the left-hand side of the page, and make ruled columns for each of those entries. Put the six exchange groups on the top of the right-hand side, and make ruled columns for each of those entries. Leave a line across the bottom for your totals.

1400-CALORIE CALCIUM KEY EXCHANGE SYSTEM FOOD DIARY
Exchanges: 4 B/G, 3 M/P, 4 V, 3 Fr, 3–4 D, 3 F

Here are the various measures you'll find in CKES:

T. = tablespoon	pc. = piece	16 oz. by weight = 1 pound
t. = teaspoon	sl. = slice	1 T. = 3 tsp.
c. = cup	(") = inches	4 T. liquid measure = ¼ c.
oz. = ounce	8 fluid oz. = 1 c. (4 fluid oz. = ½ c.)	2 T. liquid measure = 1 fluid oz.

Time	Amount	Food	B/G	M/P	V	Fr	D	F
8:30 am	¾ c.	Plain Cheerios	1					
	1 c.	Skim milk					1	
11:30 am	5	Low-fat Triscuits	1					
	1 pc.	2% American cheese singles					½	
1:15 pm	⅓ c.	White rice	1					
	1 c.	Stir-fried vegetables made with 1 t. olive oil			2			1
3:30 pm	6 oz.	Yoplait light yogurt					¾	
	1¼ c.	Strawberries				1		
5:15 pm	1	Small apple				1		
	2 t.	Peanut butter						1
8:00 pm	½ c.	Mandarin orange slices				1		
9:00 pm	1	6" Flour tortilla	1					
	3 oz.	Shredded chicken		3				
	3 T.	Shredded cheese					½	½
	1 T.	Sour cream						½
	1 c.	Cooked broccoli			2			
9:30 pm	1 c.	Skim milk					1	
TOTALS			4	3	4	3	3¾	3

2200-CALORIE CALCIUM KEY EXCHANGE SYSTEM FOOD DIARY

Exchanges: 8 B/G, 5 M/P, 6 V, 5 Fr, 3–4 D, 6 F

Time	Amount	Food	B/G	M/P	V	Fr	D	F
8:30 am	1 c.	Dannon fat-free yogurt					1	
	2 pc.	Whole-wheat toast with						
		1 T. grape jelly	2			1		
11:00 am	1	Small orange				1		
1:00 pm		1 c. iceberg lettuce, ½ c. cherry tomatoes, ½ c. broccoli, ¼ c. onions, ¼ c. carrots, 2 T. shredded cheese, 2 T. French dressing			1½		⅓	2⅓
	5	Large fried shrimp	1	1				1
	½ c.	Yellow corn (cooked in butter)	1					½
	1 c.	Cooked broccoli and cauliflower			2			
	1 c.	Cantaloupe				1		
	15	Grapes				1		
	24 oz.	Unsweetened tea						
4:00 pm	12 oz.	Diet Mountain Dew						
	6	Whole almonds						1
7:00 pm	4 oz.	Cooked ham		4				
	½ c.	Cooked green beans (cooked in fat)			1			½
	1 c.	Cooked yellow squash			2			
	1 c.	Macaroni & Cheese light	2				1	1
	16 oz.	Diet Rite soda						
9:15 pm	½	Large grapefruit				1		
10:15 pm	3	Graham cracker sheets	2					
	1 c.	1% milk					1	
		TOTALS	8	5	6½	5	3⅓	6⅓

YOUR FOOD DIARY

				Exchanges				
Time	Amount	Food	B/G	M/P	V	Fr	D	F
		TOTALS						

YOUR FOOD DIARY

| | | | | Exchanges | | | | | |
Time	Amount	Food		B/G	M/P	V	Fr	D	F
	TOTALS								

YOUR FOOD DIARY

				Exchanges					
Time	Amount	Food		B/G	M/P	V	Fr	D	F
		TOTALS							

YOUR FOOD DIARY

			Exchanges					
Time	Amount	Food	B/G	M/P	V	Fr	D	F
		TOTALS						

YOUR FOOD DIARY

| | | | | Exchanges | | | | |
Time	Amount	Food	B/G	M/P	V	Fr	D	F
		TOTALS						

YOUR FOOD DIARY

			Exchanges					
Time	Amount	Food	B/G	M/P	V	Fr	D	F
		TOTALS						

YOUR FOOD DIARY

			Exchanges					
Time	Amount	Food	B/G	M/P	V	Fr	D	F
		TOTALS						

YOUR FOOD DIARY

| | | | Exchanges | | | | | |
Time	Amount	Food	B/G	M/P	V	Fr	D	F
	TOTALS							

YOUR FOOD DIARY

| | | | | Exchanges | | | | | |
Time	Amount	Food		B/G	M/P	V	Fr	D	F
		TOTALS							

Packaged Foods: How to Read the Labels

The Combination Foods list provides some examples of foods that don't fit into any one exchange category—foods like casseroles, pizza, and soups. Many packaged foods are combination foods. The key to figuring out the exchanges in a packaged food is to match the label to the exchanges. As an example, let's look at a package of macaroni and cheese.

The top of the food label tells you the serving size and the servings in the package. With a typical package of macaroni and cheese, the serving size is 1 cup and the package contains 2 cups.

All the numerical amounts featured on the label are relevant to figuring out exchanges. And all the amounts—the Total Fat, the Total Carbohydrate, the Protein, and the Calcium—are per serving. For macaroni and cheese, a serving has 11 grams of fat. A fat exchange is 5 grams of fat. So that serving contains 2 fat exchanges.

The macaroni is pasta, which is in the bread/grains exchange category. The label says there are 31 grams of carbohydrates. A bread/grain exchange is 15 grams of carbohydrates. So that's 2 bread/grain exchanges.

You also know that macaroni and cheese includes dairy. The label says a serving supplies 20% of the Daily Value (DV) for calcium. The DV for calcium is 1000 milligrams. So a serving contains 200 milligrams of calcium. A dairy exchange has 300 milligrams of calcium. So that's two-thirds of a dairy exchange.

The total for this packaged food: 2 BG, 1 F, 2/3 D. You can go through this same process with any label.

Eating in Restaurants

With a combination food—a food that contains more than one exchange category—it's relatively easy to calculate the exchanges if you make the food at home. It's also reasonably easy with a packaged food, because you can use the numbers on the label to help you figure out exchanges. But if you eat at a restaurant, the exchanges might not be as obvious. The best way to figure out the number and type of exchanges of restaurant food is to break it down and write it down. Get in the habit of bringing your food diary with you to the restaurant.

Say you had a chicken casserole. How big was it? Did it have breading on top? How much? Did it seem to be more pasta-based or meaty? Did it have a lot of chicken in it? Did it seem like it had a lot of fat? Was the cream heavy or light?

If you ate pasta with meat sauce, how much meat was in the sauce? If you ate chili, how much was beans and how much was meat? Was the beef fatty? If you ate vegetable soup, were the vegetables starchy (bread/grain exchange) or nonstarchy (vegetable exchange)?

If you think through a restaurant meal and write down your observations, you will make accurate estimates of exchanges. Once you get used to CKES and you've eaten at a couple of different restaurants, you'll get a feel for which allow you to stick with the plan and which don't.

The Six Food Groups of CKES

Let's take a closer look at each of the six food groups in the Calcium Key Exchange System: Dairy (D), Bread/Grains (B/G), Vegetables (V), Fruits (Fr), Meat/Protein (MP), and Fats (F). We'll also look at a group of foods that is so low in calories you don't even have to list them as exchanges: Free Foods. And we'll look at groups that typically include more than one type of exchange: Combination Foods, Sweets and Sugar, Alcoholic Beverages, and Coffee Drinks.

Dairy: 3 Exchanges Every Day

Every calorie level of CKES gives you 3 dairy exchanges a day. A typical dairy exchange is

- Milk: 1 cup of skim, 1% or 2% milk (whole milk adds a fat exchange)
- Yogurt: 8 ounces of low-fat or no-fat yogurt
- Cheese: 1½ ounces of fat-free or 2% cheese (full-fat cheese adds a fat exchange)

When it comes to exchanges, milk is a pretty straightforward food. But there are many different types of yogurt, and some add nondairy exchanges to your food budget. For sweetened yogurt, add a fruit exchange. For fruit flavoring, add a fruit exchange. For yogurt made with whole milk, add a fat exchange.

Some participants in weight loss studies at the University of Tennessee found yogurt a particularly convenient way to get their dairy exchanges every day. "Yogurt was the easiest way for me to get my dairy exchanges," says Judith, a 35-year-old salesperson who lost 22 pounds on the diet. "I timed my yogurts to my energy level and my hunger. I would typically have a yogurt on the way to work, another at midmorning, and another midafternoon. I just got on that routine and stuck with it. I eat a fruit-flavored, fat-free variety. And I love all the different flavors—raspberry, apricot-mango, blackberry, you name it."

Cheese offers you a choice of reduced or full fat. We've found that many people prefer the full-fat variety. If you choose full fat, 1½ ounces of cheese is 1 dairy and 1 fat exchange, which means you won't have a fat exchange to spend on another type of food.

Are all dairy foods a good way to get your dairy exchanges? No. You have to eat 2 cups of ice cream to get a dairy exchange, and it is also 4 fat exchanges. Other dairy foods with too much fat for too little calcium include full-fat sour cream and cream cheese. And cottage cheese is actually low in calcium—it takes 4 cups to get a dairy exchange.

Remember, too, that dairy exchanges include foods you may not think about as dairy, like the cheese on pizza. Count every source of dairy, including the milk you use to make pudding, hot chocolate, or milk-based soups. You'll find a list of the calcium, calories, and fat levels of dozens of different dairy foods beginning on page 98.

A few dairy foods are fortified with calcium. That calcium does not count toward your dairy exchange. Nondairy calcium only works half as well as dairy foods in helping you shed pounds.

You can spread your spending throughout the day. Maybe you want to get 6 half exchanges rather than 3 full exchanges. Do it any way you want. That's part of the freedom and ease of the Calcium Key Weight-Loss Plan.

Breads and Grains and Starchy Vegetables

Perhaps the most important thing to notice about the breads and grains exchange list is the same thing to notice on all the exchange lists: some single *items* (like bagels) are not single *exchanges.*

One bread/grain exchange contains 15 grams of carbohydrates and 90 calories. A large, unsweetened bagel from the bagel shop is likely to contain 90 grams of carbohydrates and 540 calories. That's 6 bread/grain exchanges! A sweetened bagel is even more: 6 bread/grain and 1 fruit exchange. Similarly, a bread stick in a restaurant made with lots of butter is 2 bread/grain exchanges and 1 fat exchange.

Notice, too, that this category includes not only breads and grains but also high-carbohydrate (starchy) vegetables and legumes: corn, potatoes, squash, beans, peas, and lentils. A good rule of thumb for those foods when figuring out their exchange levels is that a half cup is 1 bread/grain exchange. However, remember that 1 cup of *cooked* beans, peas, or lentils is 1 bread/grain exchange; 1 cup of *uncooked* beans, peas, or lentils is 2 bread/grain and 1 meat/protein exchange. The uncooked cup contains enough carbohydrates and proteins to equal those extra exchanges.

You'll find that many items on the bread/grain exchange list include enough fat for 1 or even 2 fat exchanges. This is particularly true of snack chips: 15 chips, or 1 ounce, are 1 bread/grain exchange and 2 fat exchanges.

That doesn't mean you have to give up on crunchy snacks: 3 cups of low-fat popcorn are 1 bread/grain exchange. That's a lot of snacking.

If you choose low-fat versions of various foods in the bread/grain exchange category—low-fat popcorn, low-fat granola bars, low-fat chips—you'll be able to spend a fat exchange elsewhere—for example, for mayonnaise, peanut butter, salad dressing, or butter. Another smart way to save on bread/grain exchanges is to use lower-calorie bread: 2 slices of light bread are 1 bread/grain exchange rather than 2. An additional way to avoid spending a fat exchange when you eat bread is to substitute a kaiser roll, onion roll, or English muffin for biscuits or croissants. And watch out for fat-added breads, like pastries, cornbread, and muffins.

Vegetables: A Low-Cal Way to Fill Up

One vegetable exchange contains 25 calories. Another way to think about vegetable exchanges is that 1 exchange is a half cup of cooked vegetables, 1 cup of raw vegetables, or a half cup of vegetable juice. Remember that starchy vegetables, like corn, peas and potatoes, are in the bread and grains category.

You'll also find many vegetables that are 20 calories and under on the Free Foods list, such as celery, green peppers, hot peppers, mushrooms, radishes, and lettuce. You can eat as much of these vegetables as you like.

In general, we recommend that you eat bigger servings of vegetables than you have in the past—that you see veggies as a major part of your meal rather than a side dish. Vegetable-rich salads are a particularly healthy and appetite-satisfying way to achieve low-budget eating.

Cooked vegetables are best grilled or steamed without added fat. If they're cooked with fat, you'll have to add 1 or more fat exchanges, depending on the amount of fat you use.

There are many ways to get more vegetables into your diet. Put leftover vegetables into a pita or flour tortilla, add chicken or tuna and some low-fat salad dressing, and make a wrap sandwich to take to work for lunch. Have two different kinds of vegetables at the same meal—salad and a cooked veggie or squash and broccoli. Buy precut, frozen vegetable mixes and heat them up for lunch, or stir-fry them with seasonings for dinner. You can use a cooking spray to grease the pan. Cut up fresh peppers, onions, squash, broccoli, and other vegetables and marinate them or sprinkle them with seasoning. Cut up green, red, and yellow peppers to take to work as a snack; dip them in low-fat salad dressing. Keep raw carrots and tomatoes with you for a snack or to eat along with a sandwich. Use salsa as a veggie: 5 tablespoons of salsa is 1 vegetable exchange. Get your lunch or supper from a grocery store salad bar.

Fruits: Get the Nutrition But Hold the Calories

All fruits are not created equal. A fruit exchange is 15 grams of carbohydrates and 60 calories. A large apple—4 inches across, rather than 2—is about 120 calories and counts as 2 fruit exchanges. Bananas, because they're so high in natural sugar, also count as 2 fruit exchanges. So do mangoes.

Fruit juices pack a lot of calories. Just 4 ounces of orange juice is 1 fruit exchange. It's better to eat the orange. Fruit packed in syrup is packed in extra calories: it costs you an additional half exchange. Choose canned fruits that are packed in water or in their own juice.

Dried fruits are very concentrated: very small portions are 1 exchange. Some dried fruits are prepared with oil (read the label) and will cost you as many as 2 fat exchanges.

Think, too, about what else is in the fruit. Does that baked apple include butter and sugar? If so, add 1 fat and 1 fruit exchange. Try to spend your fruit exchanges on fruit.

In CKES, a pack of M&Ms is 2 fruit exchanges and 3 fat exchanges—those sweets have the carbohydrate and fat equivalents of that number of fruit and fat exchanges. But M&Ms aren't fruit! In terms of satisfying your appetite and regulating your blood sugar, you'd be much better off to spend those 2 fruit exchanges on 2 tangerines and a cup of honeydew melon.

If you're like most North Americans, you don't eat a lot of high-fiber, appetite-satisfying, nutrient-rich fruit every day. Don't think just about fresh fruit—canned and frozen are fine. Put fruit in your smoothie (see recipes in chapter 5). Keep fruit with you in the car or even in your purse. Keep fruit visible and accessible—have a fruit bowl in your kitchen or on your desk at work. Have a fruit salad with meals. Have fruit as a side dish rather than chips or fries. Have fruit on your cereal. Have fruit in your green salads; good choices include mandarin oranges, strawberries, and raisins. Bake fruits like apples and pears for tasty desserts; sweeten with Splenda (a no-calorie sweetener) and cinnamon.

Meat/Protein: Why Prime Isn't Always Best

A meat/protein exchange contains 7 grams of protein and 5 grams of fat. An exchange is 1 ounce of meat (with the exception of shellfish, where 1 exchange is 2 ounces). An ounce is about the size of a sausage patty. Peanut butter, roasted peanuts, and roasted sunflower seeds are in this exchange group. So is 4% cottage cheese, which is high in protein. To estimate servings of meat, use the visual equivalents discussed in the section earlier in this chapter, "Picturing Portions." A food scale is also very helpful.

On the exchange list, meats are organized by "best choices"—the best being meats lower in fat. That isn't because fat is bad. It's best because it doesn't include a fat exchange that you can spend on something else.

Meats that include a fat exchange are beef: prime cuts of beef, ribs, and corned beef; pork: spareribs, ground pork, and pork sausage; chicken: fried chicken or chicken with skin; fish: fried fish; cold cuts and other prepared meats: luncheon meat, sausage, knockwurst, or bratwurst. Hot dogs have 2 fat exchanges, except for turkey dogs, which have 1. Eat these high-fat meats no more than three times per week.

If you add oil or butter while preparing the meat, add a fat exchange. And if you add fat to gravy, add a fat exchange. Don't fry meats. If you pan fry, use a cooking spray. Or pan fry meats in fat-free chicken broth and seasonings. For barbeque meats, try tenderloins instead of ribs. Try chicken tenderloins with buffalo sauce instead of barbecued wings. You won't find bacon in the meat/protein section because it's almost all fat and very little protein. It's listed in the fat exchanges. A slice of bacon is 1 fat exchange.

Fat: A Little Goes a Long Way

One fat exchange contains 5 grams of fat and about 45 calories. All the servings on the list are equal to 1 exchange. To save on fat exchanges when cooking, use a cooking spray rather than oil.

Watch out for fat. Very small quantities can turn into a lot of exchanges. One-eighth of a medium avocado is 1 fat exchange, which means an entire avocado is 8 exchanges! Two tablespoons of a low-fat salad dressing is 1 exchange—pour a whole lot of that dressing on a salad, and you can quickly use up your 3 to 6 daily exchanges. You need to be even more cautious with oil: 1 teaspoon is 1 exchange. A tablespoon of cream cheese is 1 fat exchange. A teaspoon of butter is 1 fat exchange. You get the idea.

Consistently choose reduced-fat or fat-free substitutes for high-fat products. Go for low-fat sour cream, low-fat salad dressing, and low-fat mayonnaise.

The Other Exchange Lists: Free Foods, Combination Foods, Sweets and Sugar, Alcoholic Beverages, and Coffee Drinks

Let's look at the exchange lists that are not part of the six food groups in CKES.

Free Foods: Very few foods have no calories. But all the foods in the Free Foods category come close. They have 20 or fewer calories per serving.

You can eat as much as you like of free foods that don't list portion sizes—they cost nothing in your food budget. That includes vegetables like celery, lettuce, and mushrooms, beverages like club soda and black coffee, sugar-free hard candy, and a variety of condiments and seasonings.

Some free foods do list portion sizes. If you eat more than that amount, you have to list them as 1 exchange, such as ketchup (1 V), fat-free sour cream (1 F), and sugar-free pancake syrup (1 Fr).

"I loved the free food," says Phyllis, a 36-year-old mother of three, owner of a day care center, and a participant in our weight-loss studies at the University of Tennessee. "I would put a whole bunch of sliced cucumbers and a small container of low-fat salad dressing in a lunchbox and take that with me to work so I could munch something whenever I felt hungry."

Combination Foods: These include pizza, soups, and chili. Their ingredients cover more than one food group. To figure out how to calculate exchanges for combination foods, read the section called "Packaged Foods" that appears earlier in this chapter.

Sweets and Sugar: In CKES, no food is off-limits. But sweets and sugar can cost you a lot of exchanges that might be better spent elsewhere. Yes, you can have a pack of Starburst candies—for 4 fruit exchanges. Yes, you can have a 16-ounce soft drink—for 4 fruit exchanges. Yes, you can have a slice of pecan pie—for 2 bread exchanges, 2 fruit exchanges, and 4 fat exchanges.

Figure out how many grams of carbohydrates and fat are in each dessert or snack and how these fit into your daily food budget. You have to decide where and when you want to spend the exchanges. If you want the dessert, go for it. Just make sure you don't go over your exchanges for the day.

Alcoholic Beverages: Alcohol has 7 calories per gram—almost as much as fat (9 calories per gram). That means you can chug a lot of calories without too much thought. So think before you drink.

You'll see that various drinks have been broken down into exchanges based on their calorie content and contents: beer is 1 bread/grain and 1 fruit exchange; a Bloody Mary is 1 fruit, 1 vegetable, and 2 fat exchanges. You'll notice that two alcoholic beverages—light beer and wine coolers— give you a choice of exchanges. Light beer, for example, is 1 bread/grain exchange *or* 1½ fruit exchanges. This is to help you manage your daily exchanges. For example, you may have eaten your bread/grain exchanges for the day but really want a light beer with dinner. Count the beer as 1½ fruit exchanges. Options are also given in the Sweets and Sugar section for Oreo cookies.

Coffee Drinks: The calories in coffee drinks can also creep up on you, which is why they're listed in their own category. But the most important fluid in your diet isn't on this list: water. You should consume eight 8-ounce glasses of water a day. CKES includes a lot of high-fiber foods. To provide its digestion-soothing bulk, fiber needs water to expand. So drink plenty of water as part of this eating plan.

Food Exchanges for the Calcium Key Exchange System

Read through the exchange abbreviations list on page 60 daily. The more familiar you are with the food exchanges in CKES, the easier it will be to follow the plan.

Dairy (D)

One dairy exchange contains 300 milligrams (mg) of calcium and approximately 130 calories, depending on whether you choose no-fat, reduced-, or full-fat milk.

	Portion	Exchanges
Low-Fat Milk/Dairy		
Skim, 1%, or 2% milk	1 c.	1 D
Low-fat buttermilk	1 c.	1 D
Evaporated skim milk	½ c.	1 D
Dry nonfat milk	⅓ c.	1 D
Plain nonfat or low-fat yogurt	1 c.	1 D
Nonfat or low-fat artificially sweetened flavored yogurt	1 c.	1 D
Nonfat or low-fat sugar-sweetened flavored yogurt	1 c.	1 D + 1 Fr
Fat-free or 2% cheeses	1½–2 oz.	1 D
Whole Milk/Dairy		
Whole milk	1 c.	1 D + 1 F
Evaporated whole milk	½ c.	1 D + 1 F
Whole plain yogurt	1 c.	1 D + 1 F
Whole artificially sweetened flavored yogurt	1 c.	1 D + 1 F
Whole sugar-sweetened flavored yogurt	1 c.	1 D + 1 Fr + 1 F
Natural cheese (e.g., cheddar, Monterey Jack, Swiss, Colby, etc.)	1½ oz.	1 D + 1 F
Processed cheese	2 oz.	1 D + 1 F

Breads and Grains (B/G)

One bread exchange contains 15 grams of carbohydrates and 90 calories.

Breads and Grains	Portion	Exchanges
Breads		
Bagel, large unsweetened from coffee or bagel shop	1	6 B/G
Bagel, small (e.g., Original frozen Lenders' bagels)	1	2 B/G
Bagel, sweetened dessert-type from coffee or bagel shop (e.g., Panera Cinnamon Crunch)	1	6 B/G + 1 Fr
Bread/pretzel-type sticks, crisp (4–5" long × ½" wide)	2	1 B/G

Breads and Grains	Portion	Exchanges
Breads (continued)		
Biscuit, canned (Pillsbury type)	1 biscuit (2½" across)	1 B/G
Biscuit, frozen (Pillsbury type)	1 biscuit (3½" across)	1 B/G + 1 F
Chips, baked (e.g., Baked Lays, Baked Doritos, etc.)	15 chips (or 1 oz. bag)	1½ B/G
Croutons, low-fat	½ c.	1 B/G
Dinner breads (small dinner roll, small slice Italian or French, etc.)	1 sl.	1 B/G
English muffin	1	2 B/G
Hamburger/hot dog bun	1	2 B/G
Muffin, plain small (from mix made with milk)	1	1 B/G
Pita, 6" across	1	2 B/G
Raisin bread, unfrosted	1 sl.	1 B/G
Sandwich bread (white, wheat, rye, etc.)	1 sl.	1 B/G
Sandwich bread, light	2 sl.	1 B/G
Soft-baked restaurant bread sticks	1	1 B/G
Tortilla, 10" across	1	2 B/G + 1 F
Tortilla, 6" across	1	1 B/G

Cereals, Grains, and Pasta

	Portion	Exchanges
Bran cereals, concentrated (e.g., Bran Buds, All Bran, Fiber One)	⅓ c.	1 B/G
Bulgur (cooked)	½ c.	1 B/G
Cooked cereals (plain or unsweetened oatmeal, Cream of Wheat, cooked grits, etc.)	½ c.	1 B/G
Cooked cereals, sweetened (e.g., individual packets of Quaker oatmeal)	1 packet	1 B/G + 1 Fr
Granola	¼ c.	1 B/G + 1 F
Grape Nuts cereal	½ c.	3 B/G
Pasta (cooked)	½ c.	1 B/G
Rice, white or brown (cooked)	⅓ c.	1 B/G
Shredded wheat	½ c.	1 B/G
Sweetened cereals, ready to eat (e.g., Frosted Flakes, Honey Nut Cheerios, Froot Loops, etc.)	½ c.	1 B/G
Unsweetened cereals, ready to eat (e.g., Special K, Corn Flakes, plain Cheerios, Bran Flakes, etc.)	¾ c.	1 B/G
Wheat germ	3 T.	1 B/G

Dried Beans, Peas, and Lentils

	Portion	Exchanges
Beans and peas (cooked), such as kidney, white, split, black-eyed	⅓ c.	1 B/G
Lentils (cooked)	⅓ c.	1 B/G
(Note: 1 c. of beans or lentils counts as 2 breads and 1 meat.)		
Baked beans	¼ c.	1 B/G

Breads and Grains	Portion	Exchanges
Miscellaneous		
Flour	¼ c.	1 B/G
Starchy Vegetables		
Corn	½ c.	1 B/G
Corn on cob, 6" long	1 ear	1 B/G
Lima beans	½ c.	1 B/G
Peas, green (canned or frozen)	½ c.	1 B/G
Plantain	½ c.	1 B/G
Potato, baked (small: the size of a tennis ball)	1 potato	1 B/G
Potato, mashed	½ c.	1 B/G
Squash, winter (acorn, butternut)	¾ c.	1 B/G
Yam/sweet potato (plain)	⅓ c.	1 B/G
Crackers and Snacks		
Graham crackers, 2½-inch square (1½ sheets)	3 squares	1 B/G
Melba toast	5 sl.	1 B/G
Oyster crackers	24 crackers	1 B/G
Popcorn, low-fat	3 c. popped	1 B/G
Saltine-type crackers	6 crackers	1 B/G
Whole-wheat crackers, no fat added (crisp breads such as Finn, Kavli, Wasa)	2–4 crackers	1 B/G
Biscuit, fast food (e.g., Hardee's)	1 biscuit	3 B/G + 2 F
Biscuit, restaurant (e.g., Cracker Barrel)	1 biscuit (2½" across)	1 B/G + 1 F
Chow mein noodles	½ c.	1 B/G + 1 F
Cornbread, 2" cube	1 cube	1 B/G + 1 F
Cracker, round butter-type (e.g., Ritz)	6 crackers	1 B/G + 1 F
French fried potatoes (2–3½" long)	10 fries	1 B/G + 1 F
Store/bakery-bought muffin (e.g., Otis Spunkmeyer)	1 muffin	2 B/G + 2 F
Pancake, 4" across	3 pancakes	2 B/G + 1 F
Stuffing, bread (prepared)	¼ c.	1 B/G + 1 F
Taco shell, 6" across	2 shells	1 B/G + 1 F
Frozen waffle, 4½" square (e.g., Eggo) (Note: Do not count a fat exchange for low-fat varieties.)	2 waffles	2 B/G + 1 F
Whole-wheat crackers, fat added (e.g., Triscuits)	4–6 crackers	1 B/G + 1 F
Granola bar (Note: Do not count a fat exchange for low-fat varieties.)	1 small bar	1 B/G + 1 F
Snack chips (potato chips, corn chips, tortilla chips, etc.)	15 chips (or 1 oz. bag)	1 B/G + 2 F
Popcorn, regular fat	3 c. popped	1 B/G + 2 F

Vegetables (nonstarchy) (V)

One vegetable exchange contains 25 calories. Unless otherwise noted, the serving size for 1 vegetable exchange is a half cup of cooked vegetables, a half cup of vegetable juice, or 1 cup of raw vegetables.

Artichoke (½ medium)
Asparagus
Beans (green, waxed, Italian)
Bean sprouts
Beets
Broccoli
Brussels sprouts
Cabbage, cooked
Carrots
Cauliflower
Cucumber
Eggplant
Greens (turnip, mustard, collard)
Kohlrabi
Leeks

Mushrooms, cooked
Okra
Onions
Pea pods
Peppers (sweet, green, or colored)
Romaine lettuce and other dark leafy greens
Rutabaga
Sauerkraut
Spinach
Summer squash (yellow crookneck)
Tomato (1 large)
Tomato/vegetable/V-8 juice
Turnips
Water chestnuts
Zucchini, cooked

Fruits (Fr)

One fruit exchange contains 15 grams of carbohydrates and 60 calories.

Fruits	Portion	Exchanges
Fresh, Frozen, and Canned Fruits		
Apple, raw, 2" across	1 whole	1 Fr
Applesauce, unsweetened or in its own juice	½ c.	1 Fr
Apricots, medium, raw	4 whole	1 Fr
Apricots, canned (unsweetened)	½ c. or 4 halves	1 Fr
Banana (9" long)	1	2 Fr
Blackberries, raw	¾ c.	1 Fr
Blueberries, raw	¾ c.	1 Fr
Cantaloupe, 5" across	⅓ melon	1 Fr
Cantaloupe, cubes	1 c.	1 Fr
Cherries, large, raw	12	1 Fr
Cherries, canned (unsweetened)	½ c.	1 Fr
Fruit cocktail, canned (unsweetened)	½ c.	1 Fr
Grapefruit, medium	½	1 Fr
Grapefruit, sections	¾ c.	1 Fr
Grapes, small	15	1 Fr
Honeydew melon, medium	⅛ melon	1 Fr

Fruits	Portion	Exchanges
Fresh, Frozen, and Canned Fruits (continued)		
Honeydew melon, cubes	1 c.	1 Fr
Kiwi, large	1 whole	1 Fr
Mandarin oranges (unsweetened)	¾ c.	1 Fr
Mango, small	1	2 Fr
Nectarine, 1½" across	1 whole	1 Fr
Orange, 2½" across	1 whole	1 Fr
Papaya	1 c.	1 Fr
Peach, 2¾" across	1 whole or ¾ c.	1 Fr
Peaches, canned (unsweetened)	½ c. or 2 halves	1 Fr
Pear	½ large or 1 small	1 Fr
Pears, canned (unsweetened)	½ c. or 2 halves	1 Fr
Persimmon, medium, native	2 whole	1 Fr
Pineapple, raw	¾ c.	1 Fr
Pineapple, canned (unsweetened)	⅓ c.	1 Fr
Plum, raw, 2" across	2 whole	1 Fr
Pomegranate	1	2 Fr
Raspberries, raw	1 c.	1 Fr
Strawberries, raw, whole	1¼ c.	1 Fr
Tangerine, 2½" across	2 whole	1 Fr
Dried Fruit		
Apples	4 rings	1 Fr
Apricots	7 halves	1 Fr
Dates, medium	2½	1 Fr
Figs	1½	1 Fr
Prunes, medium	3	1 Fr
Raisins	2 T.	1 Fr
Banana chips	1 oz.	1 Fr + 2 F
(Note: Add 2 fats for bananas and other fruit mix that is prepared with oil.)		
Fruit Juice		
Apple juice/cider	½ c.	1 Fr
Cranberry juice cocktail	⅓ c.	1 Fr
Grapefruit juice	⅓ c.	1 Fr
Grape juice	⅓ c.	1 Fr
Juice blends (e.g., Juicy Juice, Ocean Spray Cran-Grape, etc.)	½ c.	1 Fr
Orange juice	½ c.	1 Fr
Pineapple juice	½ c.	1 Fr
Prune juice	⅓ c.	1 Fr

Meat and Protein (M/P)

One meat/protein exchange contains 7 grams of protein and 5 grams of fat, and approximately 130 calories, depending on whether the meat is lean or high in fat. Each portion is equal to 1 meat exchange.

Meat and Protein	Portion
Beef	
Best choices:	1 oz.
USDA Good or Choice grades of lean beef (round, sirloin, and flank steak)	
Tenderloin	
Chipped beef	
Next best choices:	1 oz.
Ground beef	
Roast (rib, chuck, rump)	
Steak (cubed, Porterhouse, T-bone)	
Meatloaf	
Add a fat exchange for the beef cuts listed below.	1 oz.
Most USDA Prime cuts of beef: ribs, corned beef	
Pork	
Best choices:	1 oz.
Fresh ham	
Canned, cured, or boiled ham	
Canadian bacon	
Tenderloin	
Next best choices:	1 oz.
Chops	
Loin roast	
Boston butt	
Cutlets	
Add a fat exchange for the pork cuts listed below:	1 oz.
Spareribs	
Ground pork	
Pork sausage (patty or link)	
Veal	
Best choices:	1 oz.
Chops	
Roasts	
Next best choices:	1 oz.
Cutlets: ground or cubed, unbreaded	
Poultry	
Best choices:	1 oz.
Chicken	

Meat and Protein	Portion

Poultry (continued)

Turkey
Cornish hen
Ground chicken or turkey breast · 1 oz.
Next best choices:
Domestic duck or goose
Ground turkey · 1 oz.
Add a fat exchange for the chicken cuts listed below:
Chicken with skin or any fried chicken product

Fish

Best choices:
All fresh and frozen fish · 1 oz.
Crab, lobster, scallops, or clams (fresh or canned in water) · 2 oz.
Shrimp (without breading or fat) · 5 large
Oysters, medium · 6
Water-packed tuna · ¼ c.
Next best choices: · ¼ c.
Tuna canned in oil (drained)
Add a fat exchange for any fried fish product. · 1 oz.

Wild Game

Best choices:
Venison, rabbit, pheasant, duck, or goose (skinless) · 1 oz.

Other

Best choices:
95% fat-free luncheon meat · 1 oz.
Egg whites · 3
Egg substitutes with less than 55 calories per ¼ cup · ¼ c.
Low-fat frankfurter (e.g., Healthy Choice) · 1
Fat-free or 1% cottage cheese · ¼ c.
Next best choices:
86% fat-free luncheon meat · 1 oz.
2% cottage cheese · ¼ c.
Egg (high in cholesterol—limit to 3 per week) · 1
Egg substitutes with 56–80 calories per ¼ c. · ¼ c.
Tofu (2½ inches × 2¾ inches × 1 inch) · 4 oz.
Boiled soybeans · ¼ c.
Roasted soybeans · 2 T.
Add a fat exchange for the products listed below:
Regular luncheon meat (bologna, salami, pimiento loaf) · 1 oz.
4% cottage cheese · ¼ c.
Sausage (Polish, Italian) · 1 oz.
Knockwurst (smoked) or bratwurst · 1 oz.

Meat and Protein	Portion
Other (continued)	
Frankfurter (turkey)	1 frank
Frankfurter (beef, pork, or combination)—*Add 2 fat exchanges for these*	1 frank
Peanut butter—*Add 2 fat exchanges for 2 T*	2 T.
Note: 1 T. = ½ M/P, 1 fat	
1–2 t. = 0 M/P, 1 fat	
Roasted peanuts	3 T.
Roasted sunflower seeds	¼ c.

Fats (F)

One fat exchange contains 5 grams of fat and about 45 calories. Each portion listed below is equal to 1 fat exchange.

Fats	Portion
Unsaturated Fats (Healthier)	
Avocado	⅛ medium
Guacamole	2 T.
Light/low-fat salad dressing (see "Free Foods" list for fat-free and low-cal dressing)	2 T.
Low-fat/light margarine (trans-fatty acid free)	1 T.
Low-fat/light mayonnaise	1 T.
Mayonnaise	1 t.
Oil (any type)	1 t.
Olives	10 small or 5 large
Regular salad dressing	1 T.
Nuts	
Almonds	6 whole
Cashews	1 T.
Other nuts	1 T.
Peanuts	20 small or 10 large
Pecans	2 whole
Walnuts	2 whole
Seeds	
Pine nuts	1 T.
Pumpkin seeds	2 t.
Sunflower seeds (no shells)	1 T.
Saturated Fats (limit if possible)	
Bacon	1 sl.
Bacon grease	1 t.
Beef suet	¼ oz.
Butter	1 t.

Fats	Portion
Saturated Fats (limit if possible) (continued)	
Chitterlings	½ oz.
Coconut, shredded	2 T.
Coffee creamer, liquid	2 T.
Coffee creamer, powdered	4 t.
Cream cheese	1 T.
Fatback	1 t.
Heavy whipping cream	1 T.
Lard	1 t.
Pork jowl	¼ oz.
Salt pork	¼ oz.
Shortening	1 t.
Sour cream (see "Free Foods" for fat-free and light sour cream)	2 T.

Free Foods

Free foods have less than 20 calories per serving. Those with portion sizes listed should be limited to 2 or 3 servings per day. The other foods can be eaten in unlimited amounts.

Condiments
Horseradish
Ketchup (1 T.)
Mustard
Pickles
Salad dressing, low-calorie,
    fat-free (2 T.)
Taco sauce (1 T.)
Vinegar
Fat-free or light sour cream
    (1 T.)

Drinks
Bouillon, fat-free broth
Carbonated drinks, sugar-free
Carbonated water
Club soda
Cocoa powder, unsweetened
    (1 T.)
Coffee/tea
Drink mixes, sugar-free
    (e.g., Crystal Lite, etc.)
Tonic water, sugar-free

Sweet Substitutes
Hard candy, sugar-free
Gelatin, sugar-free
Gum, sugar-free
Jam/jelly, sugar-free (2 t.)
Pancake syrup, sugar-free (1–2 T.)
Sugar substitutes (e.g., Sweet & Low,
    Equal, Splenda, etc.)
Whipped topping (2 T.)

Seasonings
Basil (fresh)
Celery seeds
Chili powder
Chives
Cinnamon
Curry
Dill
Garlic
Garlic powder
Herbs
Hot pepper sauce (e.g., tabasco)
Lemon, lemon juice

Fruits
Cranberries, unsweetened
Rhubarb, unsweetened (½ c.)

Nonstick Cooking Spray
Spray for 1–2 seconds

Vegetables
Celery
Green onion (scallion)
Hot peppers
Mushrooms
Radishes
Iceberg lettuce

Lemon pepper
Lime, lime juice
Mint
Onion powder
Oregano
Paprika
Pepper
Pimiento
Salt, flavored salts (caution: high in sodium)
Soy sauce (caution: high in sodium)
Wine, used in cooking (¼ c.)
Worcestershire sauce
Flavoring extracts: vanilla, almond, walnut, peppermint, lemon, butter, etc.

Combination Foods

These combination foods do not fit into only one food list. This is a list of average values for some typical combination foods; specific brands or recipes can vary greatly.

Combination Foods	Portion	Exchanges
Casseroles, homemade	1 c.	2 B/G + 2 M/P + 1 F
Chili with beans (canned)	1 c.	2 B/G + 2 M/P + 2 F
Chow mein (without noodles or rice)	2 c.	1 B/G + 2 M/P + 2 V
Fried green tomatoes	1 tomato (4–6 slices)	1 B/G + 1 V + 1 F
Lasagna	1 c.	2 B/G + 1 M/P + 1 D + 1 F
Macaroni and cheese	1 c.	2 B/G + 1 D + 2 F
Pizza, cheese*	2 sl. of a 14"	4 B/G + 1 D + 2 F
Pizza, meat*	2 sl. of a 14"	4 B/G + 1 D + 4 F
Soups:		
Bean	1 c.	1 B/G + 1 M/P + 1 V
Chunky, all varieties	10¾-ounce can	1 B/G + 1 M/P + 1 V
Cream, made with water	1 c.	½ B/G + 1 F
Cream, 98% fat-free, made with water	1 c.	1 B/G
Cream, 98% fat-free, made with milk	1 c.	1 B/G + ½ D
Vegetable	1 c.	1 B/G
Spaghetti and meatballs	1 c.	2 B/G + 1 M/P + 1 F

*Pizza: Decrease bread servings for thin crust and increase for deep-dish.

Sweets and Sugar

Sweets and Sugar	Portion	Exchanges
Cake/Pie/Baked Desserts		
Angel food cake	$\frac{1}{12}$ of cake	2 B/G
Brownie (prepared from mix)	2" square	1 B/G + 1 Fr + 1 F
Cake, no frosting	$\frac{1}{12}$ of cake, or a 3" square	2 B/G + 2 F
Cake, with frosting (basic vanilla/ chocolate cake)	$\frac{1}{12}$ of cake, or a 3" square	2 B/G + 1 Fr + 1 F
Carrot cake, with icing	$\frac{1}{12}$ of cake, or a 3" square	1 B/G + 2 Fr + 6 F
Cheesecake	$\frac{1}{8}$ of pie	1 B/G + 1 Fr + 7 F
Cupcake, with icing	1	1 B/G + 1 Fr + 1 F
Fruit-filled pie	$\frac{1}{8}$ of pie	1 B/G + 1 Fr + 3 F
Pecan pie	$\frac{1}{8}$ of pie	2 B/G + 2 Fr + 4 F
Cookies		
Animal Crackers (unfrosted)	8	1 B/G
Chips Ahoy chocolate chip cookies	2	1 B/G + 2 F
Chocolate chip cookie (made from dough)	1 small (2" across)	1 B/G + 1 F
Fig Newtons	2	1 B/G + $\frac{1}{2}$ F
Gingersnaps	3	1 B/G
Little Debbie Snack Cakes	1 pack (2 cakes)	1 B/G + 2 Fr + 3 F
Oatmeal cookie	2 small	1 B/G + 1 F
Oreo cookies	2	1 B/G + 1$\frac{1}{2}$ F or 1$\frac{1}{2}$ Fr + 1$\frac{1}{2}$ F
Sugar cookies	2 small	1$\frac{1}{2}$ Fr + 1 F
Vanilla wafers	6 small	1 B/G + 1 F
Candy		
Butterfinger	1 regular-size bar	1 B/G + 2 Fr + 2 F
Candy corn	$\frac{1}{4}$ c.	3 Fr
Hershey Bar	1 regular-size bar	1$\frac{1}{2}$ Fr + 3 F or 1 B/G + 3 F
M&Ms (plain)	1 regular-size bag	2$\frac{1}{2}$ Fr + 2 F
M&Ms Peanut	1 regular-size bag	2 Fr + 3 F
Reese's Peanut Butter Cups	2	1 B/G + 1 Fr + 3 F
Skittles	1 regular-size bag	1 B/G + 3 Fr
Snickers	1 regular-size bar	1 B/G + 1 Fr + 3 F
Starburst	1 regular-size pack	4 Fr
Twix	1 pack (2 bars)	1 B/G + 1 Fr + 3 F

Sweets and Sugar	Portion	Exchanges
Ice Cream/Frozen Dessert		
Premium ice cream	½ c.	2 Fr + 3 F
Ice cream	½ c.	1 Fr + 2 F
Ice cream	1 c.	2 Fr + ½ D + 2 F
Frozen yogurt	½ c.	1 Fr + 1 F
(Note: add ½ fruit for fruit varieties.)		
Frozen yogurt	1 c.	2 Fr + ½ D + 1 F
(Note: add ½ fruit for fruit varieties.)		
Other		
Barbecue sauce	2 T.	1 Fr
Hershey's chocolate syrup	2 T.	2 Fr
Icing (store-bought)	2 T.	2 Fr + 1 F
Pudding, sugar-free, made with skim milk	½ c.	½ B/G + ½ D
Pudding, regular, made with milk	½ c.	1 B/G + ½ D
Regular soft drinks	12-ounce can	3 Fr
Sugar/honey/pancake syrup/jelly	1 T. (or 3–4 t.)	1 Fr
Sweet tea, Kool-Aid, and other sweetened drinks	½ c.	1 Fr

Alcoholic Beverages

Sweets and Sugar	Portion	Exchanges
Wine	6 oz.	1½ B/G or 2½ Fr
Margarita	6 oz.	2 B/G + 2 Fr + 2½ F
Liquor	1 oz./1 shot	1½ F
Beer	12 oz.	1 B/G + 1 Fr
Light beer	12 oz.	1 B/G or 1½ Fr
Daiquiri	6 oz.	2 B/G + 1 Fr + 2 F
Wine cooler	12 oz.	2 B/G or 3 Fr
Whiskey sour	3.5 oz.	2 Fr + 1 F
Tom Collins	7.5 oz.	2 Fr + 1 F
Screwdriver	7 oz.	2 Fr + 1 F
Bloody Mary	7.5 oz.	1 Fr + 1 V + 2 F
Piña colada	6 oz.	2 B/G + 1 Fr + 2 F
Rum and soda	8 oz.	1 Fr + 2 F

Coffee Drinks

Coffee Drinks	Portion	Exchanges
Starbucks low-fat Frappuccino	1 bottle	1 Fr + 1 D
Caramel/chocolate Macchiato	12 oz.	1 Fr + 1 D + ½ F
Latte (nonfat milk, no sugar added)	12 oz.	1½ D
Cappuccino (unsweetened)	8 oz.	½ D

Coffee Drinks	Portion	Exchanges
Specialty coffee syrups	1 shot	1 Fr
Cappuccino from machine	1 c.	1½ Fr + 1 F
Cappuccino from machine	2 c.	1 B/G + 1½ Fr + ½ D + 1½ F

Alice's Story: A Perfect Wedding

Alice is a 26-year-old salesperson with a company that supplies scientific equipment to our laboratory at the University of Tennessee. At 5'7" and 140 pounds, she wasn't what you could call overweight. "My fiancé finds me quite attractive," she told me with a shy, happy smile.

Yes, Alice was getting married in two months—a church wedding with over 200 guests. But she didn't just want to look good for the groom. She wanted to walk down the aisle in her bridal gown looking *fantastic.* That's why she arranged to drop by my office for a 5-minute chat after her sales call.

Alice explained that she worked long hours. Add the stress of preparing for a big wedding, and the last thing she wanted to do right now was go on a diet. She'd heard from a coworker that she could lose some fat and maybe a couple of pounds by eating a little more dairy every day. She wanted to know if that was really true.

I assured her that our scientific studies showed it was true. I asked her about her favorite dairy food. She said it was yogurt, and I advised her to eat three 8-ounce servings of fat-free yogurt every day, substituting the 300 to 400 calories she would get from the yogurt for a few high-calorie items in her diet.

I asked her if she drank soda or ate candy bars. She told me that she didn't like coffee, but when she was on the road and needed a pick-me-up, she stopped at a fast-food drive-through and ordered a regular cola; she hated the taste of diet colas and never drank them. She had a sugary cola just about every midmorning and midafternoon. If she cut those two colas, she could cut about 400 calories a day. I suggested she substitute a serving of yogurt for each of those two sodas, adding another yogurt early in the morning or in the evening.

I didn't see Alice for another month, then we spotted each other in the hallway. She told me the "yogurt diet" was amazing. She said she'd lost some weight in the last month and that her waist was trimmer. With that same shy, happy smile, she assured me that she planned to keep eating yogurt on her honeymoon.

Making Sure You Get Enough Calcium

This section provides an extensive table of dairy foods and their calorie, fat, and calcium contents. The table contains more than 350 foods, including various types of milk (from buttermilk to whole milk), cheese (from American to Swiss), and yogurt (from Dannon to Yoplait). It's an inspiring table, because you can see that there are a lot more ways to get 3 servings of dairy a day than, for example, from drinking a glass of skim milk with every meal.

The most important use of the table, however, is to help you make sure you're following the key element of the Calcium Key Weight-Loss Plan: getting 3 exchanges of dairy a day. One dairy exchange is 300 mg of calcium. Consult the list to see if the serving of dairy you're choosing supplies around 300 mg. Most servings do, though there are some exceptions.

Note, for example, that it takes three slices of some types of cheese food to deliver 300 mg of calcium and that those three slices give you an additional fat exchange. Some cheeses are also lower in calcium than others. Camembert, for example, only supplies 165 mg of calcium per serving. Full-fat cottage cheese supplies 250 mg if you eat 2 cups. With more than 400 calories and 19 grams of fat, that's 3 additional fat exchanges. Full-fat cream cheese is also calcium-poor.

As extensive as the table is, there are dairy foods you won't find on it, like ice cream or ice milk. That's because those foods—even the low-fat varieties—deliver too many calories for too little calcium. You have to eat 2 cups of ice cream to get a dairy exchange—and that is also 4 fat exchanges. Even fat-free, sugar-free ice cream delivers 300 calories per dairy exchange—way too much to make it an everyday source of dairy while losing weight. Ice cream is also a high-glycemic-index food: it digests quickly and therefore doesn't satisfy hunger. For losing weight on CKES, it's better to use sources of dairy that are reliably healthful. This doesn't mean you shouldn't eat ice cream; it just means that you shouldn't eat it as an everyday way to get your dairy exchanges.

Likewise, there's no need to exclude full-fat cheeses; the plan doesn't view fat as an unhealthful nutrient. Just remember to add 1 or more fat exchanges to any dairy food that is 8 grams of fat or more per serving. So, for example, if you eat 1.5 ounces of cheddar cheese at 307 mg of calcium and 14 grams of fat, you'll get 1 dairy exchange and 2 fat exchanges.

With this table, the meal plans in chapter 4, and the recipes in chapter 5, you won't have any problem getting your 3 exchanges of dairy a day.

THE HIGH-DAIRY CALCIUM GUIDE

Item	Amount	Calories	Fat (grams)	Calcium (milligrams)
Milk Products				
Buttermilk	8 oz.	91	2	264
Buttermilk Sweet Cream, Dry	1 oz.	110	2	336
Dried Buttermilk	3½ T.	103	2	314
Evaporated Milk with Added Vitamin A	½ c.	169	10	329
Fat-Free Milk without Added Vitamin A	8 fl. oz.	86	0.4	301
Instant Nonfat Dry Milk with Added Vitamin A	0.3 c.	82	0.2	283
Instant Nonfat Dry Milk without Added Vitamin A	0.3 c.	81	0.2	279
LACTAID Lactose Reduced Nonfat Milk with Added Calcium	8 fl. oz.	90	1	500
Lowfat Milk, 1%	8 fl. oz.	102	3	300
Lowfat Milk, 1%, with Milk Solids	1 c.	118	3	349
Low-Sodium Whole Milk	8 oz.	149	8	246
Low-Fat Acidophilus Milk, 1%	8 fl. oz.	101	3	298
Low-Fat Buttermilk	8 fl. oz.	98	2	284
Low-Fat Milk, 1%	8 fl. oz.	102	3	300
Low-Fat Milk, 1%, Low Lactose	8 fl. oz.	103	3	303
Low-Fat Milk, 1%, with Added Protein	8 fl. oz.	118	3	349
Low-Fat Milk, 1%, with Nonfat Milk Solids	8 fl. oz.	105	2	314
Nonfat Dry Milk with Added Vitamin A	0.3 c.	145	0.3	503
Instant Nonfat Dry Milk without Added Vitamin A	0.3 c.	81	0.2	279
Nonfat Milk, Low Lactose	8 fl. oz.	86	0.4	302
Nonfat or Skim Evaporated Milk	4 fl. oz.	100	0.3	370
Nonfat, Skim or Fat-Free Milk	8 fl. oz.	86	0.4	301
Nonfat, Skim or Fat-Free Milk with Nonfat Milk Solids	8 fl. oz.	101	1	352
Nonfat, Skim, Fat-Free Milk with Added Protein	8 fl. oz.	101	1	352
ODWALLA Chocolate	8 fl. oz.	120	3	400
ODWALLA, ODWALLAMILK, Original	8 fl. oz.	100	4	400
Partly Skimmed Evaporated Milk, Undiluted, 2% Fat, Canned	½ c.	116	3	348
Producer Milk, 3.7% Milk Fat	8 fl. oz.	156	9	290
Reduced-Fat Acidophilus Milk, 2%	8 fl. oz.	122	5	298
Reduced-Fat Buttermilk, 2%	8 fl. oz.	137	5	350
Reduced-Fat Chocolate Milk, 2%	1 c.	180	5	284
Reduced-Fat Milk, 2%	8 fl. oz.	122	5	298
Reduced-Fat Milk, 2% Low Lactose	8 fl. oz.	121	5	297
Reduced-Fat Milk, 2%, with Added Nonfat Milk Solids, without Added Vitamin A	8 fl. oz.	137	5	350
Reduced-Fat Milk, 2%, with Added Protein	8 fl. oz.	137	5	350
Reduced-Fat Milk, 2%, with Milk Solids	8 fl. oz.	138	5	352
Reduced-Fat Milk, 2%, with Nonfat Milk Solids	8 fl. oz.	125	5	314

Item	Amount	Calories	Fat (grams)	Calcium (milligrams)
Milk Products (continued)				
Skim Evaporated Milk, Undiluted, 0.2% Butter Fat, Canned	4 fl. oz.	98	0.3	365
Skim Milk	8 fl. oz.	85	0.4	298
Skim Milk Powder	0.3 c.	80	0.2	277
Skim Milk, Dry	3½ T.	95	0.2	330
Sweetened Condensed Milk	0.3 c.	324	9	287
Sweetened Condensed Milk, Canned	0.3 c.	323	9	286
Whole Chocolate Milk	8 fl. oz.	208	8	280
Whole Dry Milk	0.3 c.	212	11	389
Whole Evaporated Milk	½ c.	169	10	329
Whole Evaporated Milk, Undiluted, 7.8% Butter Fat, Canned	½ c.	157	9	300
Whole Milk, 3.3%	8 fl. oz.	149	8	290
Whole Milk, 3.7%	8 fl. oz.	157	9	293
Whole Milk, Dry	¼ t.	165	9	304
Whole Milk, Pasteurized, Homogenized, 3.3% Butter Fat	1 c.	147	8	287

Cheese Products

Item	Amount	Calories	Fat (grams)	Calcium (milligrams)
Alpine Lace Reduced-Fat Cheddar Cheese	1.5 oz.	105	7	300
Alpine Lace Reduced-Fat Mozzarella Cheese	1.5 oz.	105	5	375
Alpine Lace Reduced-Fat and -Sodium Jalapeño Cheese	1.5 oz	120	9	375
Alpine Lace Reduced-Fat and -Sodium Provolone Cheese	1 oz.	70	5	350
Alpine Lace Reduced-Fat and -Sodium Swiss Cheese	1.5 oz.	135	9	375
Alpine Lace Reduced-Fat and -Sodium White American Cheese	1.5 oz.	120	9	375
Alpine Lace Reduced-Fat and -Sodium Yellow American Cheese	1.5 oz.	120	9	375
Alpine Lace Reduced-Sodium Muenster Cheese	1 oz.	110	9	300
American Cheese Food, Cold Pack	2 oz.	188	14	282
American Cheese Food, Pasteurized Process, with Disodium Phosphate	2 oz.	186	14	325
American Cheese Food, Processed	2 oz.	186	14	326
American Cheese Spread, Processed	2 oz.	165	12	319
American Cheese Spread, Pasteurized Process, with Disodium Phosphate	2 oz.	164	12	319
American Cheese, Processed	1.5 oz.	159	13	262
Arby's Slice Swiss Cheese	1.5 oz.	137	9	304
Blue Cheese	2 oz.	200	16	299
Blue Cheese, Crumbled	2 oz.	200	16	299
Brick Cheese	1.5 oz.	158	13	286
Brie Cheese	1.5 oz.	142	12	78

Item	Amount	Calories	Fat (grams)	Calcium (milligrams)
Cheese Products (continued)				
Camembert Cheese	1.5 oz.	128	10	165
Caraway Cheese	1.5 oz.	160	12	286
Cheddar Cheese	1.5 oz.	171	14	307
Cheddar Cheese Spread, Made with Skim Milk, Processed	2 oz.	107	3	318
Cheddar Cheese Spread, Processed	2 oz.	162	12	314
Cheddar Cheese, Diced	1.5 oz.	171	14	307
Cheddar Cheese, Pieces	1.5 oz.	171	14	307
Cheddar Cheese, Processed	2 oz.	186	14	326
Cheddar Cheese, Processed with Skim Milk	2 oz.	108	4	319
Cheddar Cheese, Processed, Cold Pack	2 oz.	188	14	282
Cheddar Cheese, Shredded	1.5 oz.	171	14	307
Cheez Whiz Pasteurized, Process Cheese Sauce	0.25 c.	180	14	200
Cheez Whiz Pasteurized, Process Jalapeño Pepper Cheese	0.25 c.	180	14	200
Cheez Whiz Pasteurized, Process Mild Salsa Cheese Sauce	0.25 c.	200	14	200
Cheshire Cheese	1.5 oz.	165	13	273
Colby Cheese	1.5 oz.	165	13	288
Composite-Cheese, Cheddar/Colby/American/Monterey Jack	1.5 oz.	165	13	294
Composite-Cheese, Swiss/Mozzarella/Ricotta, Low-Fat	1.5 oz.	109	7	267
Cottage Cheese with Fruit, Creamed	2 c.	560	15	215
Cottage Cheese, <0.1% Butter Fat	2 c.	407	0.4	149
Cottage Cheese, 1% Butter Fat	2 c.	339	5	284
Cottage Cheese, 2% Butter Fat	2 c.	407	9	310
Cottage Cheese, 4.5% Butter Fat, Creamed	2 c.	433	19	252
Cottage Cheese, 4% Fat, Creamed	2 c.	433	19	252
Cottage Cheese, Dry Curd, 0.4% Butter Fat	2 c.	247	1	92
Cracker Barrel 2% Milk Natural Reduced-Fat Cheddar Cheese, Sharp	1.5 oz.	135	9	300
Cracker Barrel Whipped Spreadable Extra Sharp Cheddar Cheese, Sharp	0.25 c.	160	16	160
Cracker Barrel Whipped Spreadable Sharp Cheddar & Cream Cheese	0.25 c.	160	16	160
Cream Cheese	2 T.	101	10	23
Dorman's Deli Light Swiss Cheese, No Salt	1.5 oz.	150	12	410
Dorman's Low-Sodium Cheddar Jack Cheese	1.5 oz.	120	8	300
Dorman's Low-Sodium Monterey Cheese	1.5 oz.	120	8	300
Dorman's Low-Sodium Mozzarella Cheese	1.5 oz.	120	6	312
Dorman's Low-Sodium Muenster Cheese	1.5 oz.	120	8	306
Dorman's Low-Sodium Provolone Cheese	1.5 oz.	120	6	300
Dorman's Low-Sodium, Low-Fat Cheddar Cheese	1.5 oz.	120	8	300

Item	Amount	Calories	Fat (grams)	Calcium (milligrams)
Cheese Products (continued)				
Dorman's Low-Sodium, Low-Fat Swiss Cheese	1.5 oz	135	8	410
Easy Cheese American Pasteurized Process Cheese Spread	0.25 c.	200	14	300
Easy Cheese Cheddar 'n Bacon Pasteurized Process Cheese Spread	0.25 c.	200	14	300
Easy Cheese Cheddar Pasteurized Process Cheese Spread	0.25 c.	200	14	300
Easy Cheese Nacho Pasteurized Process Cheese Spread	0.25 c.	200	14	300
Easy Cheese Sharp Cheddar Pasteurized Process Cheese Spread	0.25 c.	200	14	300
Edam Cheese	1.5 oz.	152	12	311
Fat-Free Cream Cheese	2 T.	29	0.4	56
Feta Cheese	1.5 oz.	111	9	207
Fontina Cheese	1.5 oz.	165	13	234
Frigo Fat-Free Ricotta Cheese	0.25 c.	48	0.4	269
Frigo Low-Fat Ricotta Cheese	0.25 c.	64	2	292
Gardenia Low-Fat Ricotta Cheese	0.25 c.	65	3	243
Gjetost Cheese	1.5 oz.	198	13	170
Goat Cheese, Hard	1.5 oz.	193	15	381
Goat Cheese, Hard, <35% Water, 36% Butter Fat	1.5 oz.	194	15	384
Goat Cheese, Semisoft	1.5 oz.	155	13	127
Goat Cheese, Semisoft, 35–55% Water, 30% Butter Fat	1.5 oz.	156	13	128
Goat Cheese, Soft	1.5 oz.	114	9	60
Goat Cheese, Soft, >55% Water, 21% Butter Fat	1.5 oz.	114	9	60
Gouda Cheese	1.5 oz.	155	12	305
Gruyere Cheese	1.5 oz.	176	14	430
Handi-Snacks Low-Moisture, Part-Skim Mozzarella String Cheese	2 oz.	160	12	300
Healthy Choice Mozzarella String Cheese	1.5 oz.	75	2	300
Knudsen Free Fat-Free Cottage Cheese	2 c.	320	0	320
Kraft 2% Milk Natural Reduced-Fat Cheddar Cheese, Mild	1.5 oz.	135	9	300
Kraft 2% Milk Natural Reduced-Fat Cheddar Cheese, Sharp	1.5 oz.	135	9	300
Kraft 2% Milk Natural Reduced-Fat Colby Cheese	1.5 oz.	120	9	300
Kraft 2% Milk Natural Reduced-Fat Monterey Jack Cheese	1.5 oz.	120	9	300
Kraft 2% Milk Natural Reduced-Fat Mozzarella Cheese, Shredded	1.5 oz.	110	7	343
Kraft Deluxe Pasteurized Process American Cheese, Loaf and Chunk	2 oz.	200	18	300
Kraft Deluxe Singles Pasteurized Process American Cheese	2 oz.	220	18	300
Kraft Deluxe Singles Pasteurized Process Swiss Cheese	1.5 oz.	135	11	300

Item	Amount	Calories	Fat (grams)	Calcium (milligrams)
Cheese Products (continued)				
Kraft Free Singles Nonfat Pasteurized Process American Cheese Product Slice	2 sl.	60	0	300
Kraft Natural Cheddar Cheese, Mild	1.5 oz.	165	14	300
Kraft Natural Monterey Jack with Jalapeño Peppers Cheese	1.5 oz.	165	14	300
Kraft Pasteurized Process Cheese Food with Garlic	2 oz.	180	14	300
Kraft Pasteurized Process Cheese Food with Jalapeño Peppers	2 oz.	180	14	300
Kraft Singles Pasteurized Process American Cheese Food Slices	2 sl.	220	16	400
Kraft Singles Pasteurized Process American White Cheese Food Slices	2 sl.	140	10	200
Kraft Singles Pasteurized Process Mild Mexican Style CheeseFood Slices	2 sl.	140	10	200
Kraft Singles Pasteurized Process Monterey Cheese Food Slices	2 sl.	140	10	200
Kraft Singles Pasteurized Process Pimento Cheese Food Slices	2 sl.	120	9	200
Kraft Singles Pasteurized Process Sharp Cheese Food Slices	2 sl.	140	12	200
Kraft Singles Pasteurized Process Swiss Cheese Food Slices	2 sl.	140	10	300
Kraft Singles Sharp Cheddar Process Cheese Product, ⅓ Less Fat	2 sl.	100	6	300
Kraft Singles Swiss Process Cheese Food Slices, ⅓ Less Fat	2 sl.	100	5	300
Light N' Lively American Flavor Pasteurized Process Cheese Product Singles	2 sl.	90	5	300
Limburger Cheese	1.5 oz.	139	12	211
Low-Fat Cheddar or Colby Cheese	1.5 oz.	74	3	176
Low-Fat Cheese, 0.5% Butter Fat	1.5 oz.	23	0.2	70
Low-Fat Cottage Cheese, 1% Fat	2 c.	325	5	276
Low-Fat Cottage Cheese, 2% Fat	2 c.	407	9	312
Low-Fat Cottage Cheese, Low Lactose	2 c.	336	5	241
Low-Fat Cream Cheese	2 T.	69	5	34
Low-Fat Monterey Jack Cheese	1.5 oz.	133	9	300
Low-Fat Swiss Cheese, Shredded	1 oz.	51	1	273
Low-Sodium Cheddar or Colby Cheese	1.5 oz.	169	14	299
Low-Sodium Mozzarella Cheese, Shredded	1.5 oz.	119	7	311
Low-Sodium Muenster Cheese, Shredded	1.5 oz.	157	13	305
Low-Sodium Parmesan Cheese	2 T.	46	3	138

Item	Amount	Calories	Fat (grams)	Calcium (milligrams)
Cheese Products (continued)				
Low-Sodium Swiss Cheese, Shredded	1 oz.	107	8	273
Lucerne Fat-Free Cottage Cheese	2 c.	280	0	240
Lucerne No Salt Added 1% Fat Cottage Cheese	2 c.	320	4	240
Mexican Cheese (Queso Anejo)	1.5 oz.	159	13	289
Mexican Cheese (Queso Asadero)	1.5 oz.	151	12	281
Mexican Cheese (Queso Chihuahua)	1.5 oz.	159	13	277
Mexican Farmer Cheese (Queso Fresco	1.5 oz.	62	4	122
Monterey Jack Cheese	1.5 oz.	157	13	313
Mozzarella Cheese Substitute	1.5 oz.	106	5	260
Mozzarella Cheese, 48% Water, 25% Butter Fat	1.5 oz.	135	10	244
Mozzarella Cheese, 52% Water, 22.5% Butter Fat	1.5 oz.	125	10	230
Mozzarella Cheese, Part Skim Milk	1.5 oz.	107	7	271
Mozzarella Cheese, Part Skim Milk, Low Moisture	1.5 oz.	119	7	311
Mozzarella Cheese, Part Skim, 49% Water, 17% Butter Fat	1.5 oz.	119	7	311
Mozzarella Cheese, Part Skim, 52% Water, 16.5% Butter Fat	1.5 oz.	112	7	289
Mozzarella Cheese, Whole Milk	1.5 oz.	118	9	217
Mozzarella Cheese, Whole Milk, Low Moisture	1.5 oz.	135	10	245
Muenster Cheese	1.5 oz.	156	13	305
Neufchâtel Cheese	1 oz.	74	7	21
Nonfat Cottage Cheese, Uncreamed, Dry	0.3 c.	41	0.2	15
Parmesan Cheese, Grated	2 T.	57	4	172
Parmesan Cheese, Hard	1 oz.	111	7	336
Parmesan Cheese, Shredded	1 T.	138	9	417
Paula County Line Advantage Low-Sodium Low-Fat Swiss Cheese	1 oz.	80	4	300
Philadelphia Brand Cream Cheese with Chives, Brick	1 oz.	90	9	0
Philadelphia Brand, Cream Cheese, Brick	1 oz.	100	10	0
Philadelphia Brand Light Soft Cream Cheese	2 T.	70	5	40
Philadelphia Brand Neufchâtel Cheese	1 oz.	70	6	20
Philadelphia Brand Soft Chives and Onion Cream Cheese	2 T.	110	10	40
Philadelphia Brand Soft Cream Cheese	2 T.	100	10	20
Philadelphia Brand Soft Pineapple Cream Cheese	2 T.	100	9	40
Philadelphia Brand Soft Salmon Cream Cheese	2 T.	100	9	20
Philadelphia Brand Soft Strawberry Cream Cheese	2 T.	110	9	40
Philadelphia Brand Whipped Cream Cheese	2 T.	70	7	0
Philadelphia Brand Whipped Cream Cheese with Chives	2 T.	70	6	20
Philadelphia Brand Whipped Cream Cheese with Smoked Salmon	2 T.	70	6	20
Pimento Cheese, Processed	1.5 oz.	159	13	261

Item	Amount	Calories	Fat (grams)	Calcium (milligrams)
Cheese Products (continued)				
Port du Salut Cheese	1.5 oz.	148	12	273
Provolone Cheese	1.5 oz.	147	11	318
Reduced-Calorie Cheese, 3% Butter Fat	1.5 oz.	26	1	51
Reduced-Calorie Cheese, 6% Butter Fat	1.5 oz.	85	3	299
Reduced-Calorie Cream Cheese, 20% Butter Fat	1.5 oz.	95	8	39
Ricotta Cheese, Part Skim Milk	0.25 c.	85	5	167
Ricotta Cheese, Whole Milk	0.25 c.	107	8	127
Romano Cheese	1 oz.	110	8	302
Roquefort (Blue) Cheese	1.5 oz.	157	13	281
Roquefort Cheese	1.5 oz.	155	13	278
Sapsago Cheese	1 oz.	50	0	300
Sargento Blend Shredded 4 Cheese Mexican	1.5 oz.	167	14	304
Sargento Blend Shredded 6 Cheese Italian	1.5 oz.	137	11	304
Sargento Blend Shredded Nacho & Taco Cheese	1.5 oz.	167	14	304
Sargento Blend Shredded Parmesan & Romano Cheese	1.5 oz.	167	11	380
Sargento Blend Shredded Pizza Double Cheese	1.5 oz.	137	9	304
Sargento Blend Shredded Taco Cheese	1.5 oz.	167	14	304
Sargento Colby-Jack Cheese Sticks	1.5 pc.	165	14	300
Sargento Crumbled Blue Cheese	1.5 oz.	152	12	228
Sargento Deli Style Sliced Aged Swiss Cheese	1 sl.	70	5	200
Sargento Deli Style Sliced Colby Cheese	2 sl.	160	14	300
Sargento Deli Style Sliced Jarlsberg Cheese	1 sl.	80	6	200
Sargento Deli Style Sliced Muenster Cheese	2 sl.	160	12	300
Sargento Deli Style Sliced Monterey Jack Cheese	2 sl.	160	12	300
Sargento Deli Style Sliced Sharp Cheddar Cheese	2 sl.	160	14	300
Sargento Deli Style Thin Sliced Swiss Cheese	1 sl.	70	5	200
Sargento Deli Style Sliced Mozzarella Cheese	2 sl.	120	8	300
Sargento Fancy Shredded Colby-Jack Cheese	1.5 oz.	167	14	304
Sargento Fancy Shredded Mild Cheddar Cheese	1.5 oz.	167	14	304
Sargento Fancy Shredded Monterey Jack Cheese	1.5 oz.	167	14	304
Sargento Fancy Shredded Mozzarella Cheese	1.5 oz.	121	9	304
Sargento Fancy Shredded Parmesan Cheese	1.5 oz.	167	11	380
Sargento Fancy Shredded Swiss Cheese	1 oz.	111	8	304
Sargento Light Deli Style Sliced Mozzarella Cheese	1 sl.	60	3	200
Sargento Light Deli Style Sliced Provolone Cheese	2 sl.	90	5	300
Sargento Light Deli Style Sliced Swiss Cheese	1 sl.	70	4	250
Sargento Light Ricotta Cheese	0.25 c.	60	3	100
Sargento Light Shredded Mild Cheddar Cheese	1.5 oz.	106	7	380
Sargento Light Shredded Mozzarella Cheese	1.5 oz.	106	5	304
Sargento Light String Cheese Snacks	2 pc.	100	5	300
Sargento Mild Cheddar Cheese Sticks	1 pc.	110	9	200

Item	Amount	Calories	Fat (grams)	Calcium (milligrams)
Cheese Products (continued)				
Sargento Part Skim Ricotta Cheese	1.5 oz.	48	3	69
Sargento String Cheese Snacks	1 item	80	6	200
Sargento Whole Milk Ricotta Cheese	1.5 oz.	62	4	103
Smart Beat Fat-Free American Cheese	2 sl.	50	0	300
Smart Beat Fat-Free Sharp Cheese	2 sl.	50	0	300
Swiss Cheese	1 oz.	105	8	269
Swiss Cheese (Emmental)	1 oz.	107	8	272
Swiss Cheese Food, Processed	1.5 oz.	137	10	307
Swiss Cheese, Pasteurized Process	1.5 oz.	142	11	328
Swiss Cheese, Processed	1.5 oz.	142	11	328
Tilsit Cheese	1.5 oz.	143	11	294
Tilsit Cheese Made with Whole Milk	1.5 oz.	145	11	298
Velveeta Hot Mexican Process Cheese Food, Shredded	0.25 c.	130	9	200
Velveeta Mild Mexican Pasteurized Process Cheese Food with Jalapeño Pepper, Shredded	0.25 c.	120	9	200
Velveeta Pasteurized Process Cheese Food, Shredded	0.25 c.	130	9	200
Velveeta Pasteurized Process Hot Mexican Process Cheese Spread	1.5 oz.	135	9	225
Weight Watchers Fat-Free Swiss Cheese Slices	2 sl.	30	0	150
Weight Watchers Natural Cheddar Cheese, Mild and Sharp	1.5 oz.	120	8	300
Weight Watchers Reduced-Sodium Fat-Free Yellow Cheese Slices	2 sl.	30	0	150
Yogurt Products				
Coffee or Vanilla Flavor Yogurt, 1.9% Butter Fat	1 c.	209	4	298
Dannon Low-Fat Apple Cinnamon Yogurt	1 c.	210	2	300
Dannon Low-Fat Blueberry Yogurt	1 c.	210	2	300
Dannon Low-Fat Boysenberry Yogurt	1 c.	210	2	300
Dannon Low-Fat Cherry Yogurt	1 c.	210	2	300
Dannon Low-Fat Coffee Yogurt	1 c.	220	4	350
Dannon Low-Fat Cranberry-Raspberry Yogurt	1 c.	220	4	350
Dannon Low-Fat French Vanilla Raspberry Yogurt	1 c.	240	3	300
Dannon Low-Fat French Vanilla Strawberry Yogurt	1 c.	240	3	300
Dannon Low-Fat Lemon Yogurt	1 c.	220	4	350
Dannon Low-Fat Mixed Berries Yogurt	1 c.	210	2	300
Dannon Low-Fat Peach Yogurt	1 c.	210	2	300
Dannon Low-Fat Raspberry Yogurt	1 c.	210	2	300
Dannon Low-Fat Strawberry Banana Yogurt	1 c.	210	2	300
Dannon Low-Fat Strawberry Yogurt	1 c.	210	2	300
Dannon Low-Fat Tropical Flavor with Peaches Yogurt	1 c.	240	3	300

Item	Amount	Calories	Fat (grams)	Calcium (milligrams)
Yogurt Products (continued)				
Dannon Low-Fat Vanilla Yogurt	1 c.	230	4	350
Dannon Low-Fat Plain Yogurt	1 c.	150	4	350
Fruit Bottom Yogurt, <1% Butter Fat	1 c.	141	0.4	364
Fruit Bottom Yogurt, >4% Butter Fat	1 c.	327	14	244
Fruit Bottom Yogurt, 1–2% Butter Fat	1 c.	229	3	277
Fruit Bottom Yogurt, 2–4% Butter Fat	1 c.	261	7	324
Fruit Yogurt, Stirred or Swiss Style	1 c.	231	4	313
Light N' Lively Free Nonfat Strawberry Yogurt	4.4 oz.	70	0	100
Low-Fat Fruit Yogurt (10 grams protein per 8 oz.)	1 c.	231	2	345
Low-Fat Fruit Yogurt (11 grams protein per 8 oz.)	1 c.	238	3	383
Low-Fat Plain Yogurt (12 grams protein per 8 oz.)	1 c.	143	4	415
Low-Fat Fruit Yogurt (9 grams protein per 8 oz.)	1 c.	225	3	313
Low-Fat Vanilla Yogurt (11 grams protein per 8 oz.)	1 c.	193	3	388
McDonald's Fruit n' Yogurt Parfait	1 item	380	5	300
McDonald's Fruit n' Yogurt Parfait without granola	1 item	280	4	250
Nonfat Fruit Yogurt, Sweetened with Low-Calorie Sweetener	1 c.	115	0.4	348
Nonfat Plain Yogurt (13 grams protein per 8 oz.)	1 c.	127	0.4	451
Plain Yogurt with Whole Milk (8 grams protein per 8 oz.)	1 c.	138	7	274
Plain Yogurt, <1% Butter Fat	1 c.	116	0.2	381
Plain Yogurt, >4% Butter Fat	1 c.	236	13	342
Plain Yogurt, 2–4% Butter Fat	1 c.	161	6	365
Plain Yogurt, Stirred or Swiss Style	1 c.	154	5	413
Stonyfield Farm Nonfat Apricot Mango Yogurt	1 c.	160	0	450
Stonyfield Farm Nonfat Blueberry Yogurt	1 c.	160	0	450
Stonyfield Farm Nonfat Cappuccino Yogurt	1 c.	160	0	450
Stonyfield Farm Nonfat French Vanilla Yogurt	1 c.	160	0	450
Stonyfield Farm Nonfat Lotsa Lemon Yogurt	1 c.	160	0	400
Stonyfield Farm Nonfat Peach Yogurt	1 c.	150	0	450
Stonyfield Farm Nonfat Plain Yogurt	1 c.	100	0	450
Stonyfield Farm Nonfat Raspberry Yogurt	1 c.	160	0	450
Stonyfield Farm Organic Blended Banana Low-Fat Yogurt	6 oz.	170	2	250
Stonyfield Farm Organic Blended Peach Low-Fat Yogurt	6 oz.	170	2	250
Stonyfield Farm Organic Blended Raspberry Low-Fat Yogurt	6 oz.	160	2	250
Stonyfield Farm Organic Blended Strawberry Low-Fat Yogurt	6 oz.	170	2	250
Stonyfield Farm Organic Low-Fat Blueberry Yogurt	6 oz.	130	2	250
Stonyfield Farm Organic Low-Fat Caramel Yogurt	6 oz.	170	2	300
Stonyfield Farm Organic Low-Fat Just Peachy Yogurt	6 oz.	130	2	250

Item	Amount	Calories	Fat (grams)	Calcium (milligrams)
Yogurt Products (continued)				
Stonyfield Farm Organic Low-Fat Luscious Lemon Yogurt	6 oz.	130	2	350
Stonyfield Farm Organic Low-Fat Maple Vanilla Yogurt	6 oz.	120	2	300
Stonyfield Farm Organic Low-Fat Mocha Latte Yogurt	6 oz.	120	2	300
Stonyfield Farm Organic Low-Fat Plain Yogurt	6 oz.	80	2	300
Stonyfield Farm Organic Low-Fat Raspberry Yogurt	6 oz.	130	2	250
Stonyfield Farm Organic Low-Fat Strawberry Yogurt	6 oz.	130	2	250
Stonyfield Farm Organic Low-Fat Vanilla Yogurt	6 oz.	120	2	300
Stonyfield Farm Organic Whole-Milk Creamy Maple Yogurt	6 oz.	160	6	250
Stonyfield Farm Organic Whole-Milk French Vanilla Yogurt	6 oz.	170	6	350
Stonyfield Farm Organic Whole-Milk Mochaccino Yogurt	6 oz.	170	6	250
Stonyfield Farm Organic Whole-Milk Plain Yogurt	1 c.	180	10	450
Stonyfield Farm Organic Whole-Milk Strawberries & Cream Yogurt	6 oz.	160	5	200
Stonyfield Farm Organic Whole-Milk Vanilla Truffle Yogurt	6 oz.	220	5	250
Stonyfield Farm Organic Whole-Milk Wild Blueberry Yogurt	6 oz.	160	5	200
Weight Watchers Ultimate 90 Blueberries 'n Creme Yogurt	1 c.	90	0	250
Weight Watchers Ultimate 90 Cappuccino Yogurt	1 c.	90	0	250
Weight Watchers Ultimate 90 Cherries Jubilee Yogurt	1 c.	90	0	250
Weight Watchers Ultimate 90 Cranberry Raspberry Yogurt	1 c.	90	0	250
Weight Watchers Ultimate 90 Lemon Chiffon Yogurt	1 c.	90	0	250
Weight Watchers Ultimate 90 Peach Yogurt	1 c.	90	0	250
Weight Watchers Ultimate 90 Plain Yogurt	1 c.	90	0	300
Weight Watchers Ultimate 90 Raspberries 'n Creme Yogurt	1 c.	90	0	250
Weight Watchers Ultimate 90 Strawberry Banana Yogurt	1 c.	90	0	250
Weight Watchers Ultimate 90 Strawberry Yogurt	1 c.	90	0	250
Weight Watchers Ultimate 90 Vanilla Yogurt	1 c.	90	0	250
Yoplait 99% Fat-Free Original Yogurt, Fruit Flavors	6 oz.	170	2	200
Yoplait Custard Style Yogurt, Fruit Flavors	6 oz.	190	4	200
Yoplait Light Yogurt, Fruit Flavors	6 oz.	90	0	200
Yoplait Vanilla Custard Style Yogurt	6 oz.	190	4	200

Simple and Effective Solutions for Lactose Intolerance

Maybe you've decided that the Calcium Key Weight-Loss Plan isn't for you because the thought of consuming 3 to 4 daily servings of dairy foods makes you feel literally sick. If that's the case, you're probably among the approximately 50 million North Americans who sometimes experience one or more (usually mild) digestive symptoms—for example, gas, bloating, stomach pain, or diarrhea—after they eat or drink dairy foods.

This condition is called *lactose intolerance.*

Dairy foods contain a sugar called *lactose.* Lactose is a *disaccharide,* or double sugar; to absorb it, the body splits it into two simple sugars, galactose and glucose. The intestinal enzyme that does this job is called *lactase.* But if your gut doesn't have enough lactase, lactose isn't digested. Instead, it proceeds intact from the small intestine to the large intestine, or colon, where bacteria ferment it, generating hydrogen gas. And 30 minutes to a couple of hours after eating or drinking a lactose-containing food, the gas can cause digestive distress.

Diseases that damage the small intestine can cause lactose intolerance. So can parasitic infections and some medications. But the most common cause is genetic: in about two-thirds of the world's population, at around the age of 3 to 5, the ability to produce lactase falls by 90 to 95%. Lactose intolerance affects many Asian-Americans (90%), Native Americans (90%), African-Americans (80%), and Hispanic Americans (53%). Caucasians in the United States, particularly those of northern European descent, have the lowest rate of lactose intolerance, at 6 to 22%. Scientists speculate that in areas of the world where there was more dairy farming, like northern Europe, people developed the genetic ability to digest lactose beyond childhood.

But no matter what your ethnicity and no matter what your past experience with dairy products, you can easily, enjoyably, and healthfully go on the Calcium Key Weight-Loss Plan. Even if you have lactose intolerance, you can get your 3 to 4 servings of dairy a day *and* be virtually symptom-free. That's not my opinion, but a scientifically proven fact.

Ask yourself, "Will consuming more dairy really cause me discomfort?" This was the question asked by scientists at the Minneapolis Veterans Affairs Medical Center. In a study published in the *American Journal of Clinical Nutrition,* the scientists point out that it is widely believed that the lactose content of dairy products will not be tolerated by people with lactose intolerance. Seems obvious enough. But is it true?

To find out, the scientists tested 62 women—31 with lactose intolerance and 31 without—for 2 weeks. For 1 week, the women consumed dairy foods with lactose. For another week, they consumed dairy foods without lactose (so-called lactose-hydrolyzed products). The two types of dairy food were processed to look and taste the same so that the women couldn't tell which was which. In all, the women got daily servings of 2 cups of 1% fat milk, 2 ounces of hard cheese, and 1 cup of low-fat yogurt—about the same amount of dairy as recommended by the Calcium Key Weight-Loss Plan.

The results are good news for anyone with lactose intolerance who wants to go on CKES. While some women with lactose intolerance did experience "slightly greater" amounts of gas, say the researchers, "bloating, abdominal pain, diarrhea, and the global perception of overall symptom severity were not significantly different between the 2 treatment periods." Their conclusion: "The symptoms resulting from lactose intolerance are not a major impediment to the ingestion of a dairy-rich diet supplying approximately 1500 milligrams of calcium a day."

In another study along these lines conducted by researchers at the University of Minnesota and published in the *New England Journal of Medicine,* 30 people who described themselves as having severe lactose intolerance were given a daily 8-ounce glass of milk with or without lactose (like the previous study, they didn't know which was which). Every day, the participants reported the severity of their gastrointestinal symptoms: bloating, abdominal pain, gas, diarrhea. The result was no difference in symptoms between the days the participants got lactose and the days they didn't. The researchers concluded, "People who identify themselves as severely lactose-intolerant may mistakenly attribute a variety of abdominal symptoms to lactose intolerance."

There are many other studies of this kind on people of varying ethnic backgrounds and on the elderly. (Lactose intolerance may become worse with age, though studies are contradictory.) Most show the same result: little or no difference in digestive symptoms when groups of people who said they were lactose intolerant consumed either high-lactose or lactose-free dairy products.

Even if you think you're lactose intolerant, you may be able to increase your consumption of dairy products without an increase in symptoms. And there are a few ways to avoid symptoms altogether that may work for you. The first is to start consuming more dairy foods.

Reducing the Symptoms of Lactose Intolerance

Getting more dairy may seem like an odd way to overcome lactose intolerance, but it's not. Studies show that when you start eating dairy, the bacteria in your colon gradually adapt to the lactose, fermenting less and less.

In one study led by Dennis A. Savaiano, Ph.D., professor in the Department of Foods and Nutrition at Purdue University in Indiana, published in the *American Journal of Clinical Nutrition,* 20 people with lactose intolerance were fed increasing amounts of either a supplement of lactose or a supplement of dextrose (another sugar) for the first 10 days of the study. For days 12 to 21, the groups switched—those who had received the dextrose started receiving lactose, and vice versa. On days 11 and 22, the researchers gave all 20 people a challenge dose of lactose in the morning. Then, for the next 8 hours, the researchers measured symptoms (abdominal pain, gas, and diarrhea) and levels of hydrogen in the breath (higher levels mean there's more hydrogen in the colon, which means more lactose is fermenting).

Those who had received lactose for the previous 10 days had symptoms that were 50% milder than those who had received dextrose. Breath levels of hydrogen among people who had been given lactose most recently were much lower than among those who had been given dextrose most recently.

Why were symptoms less when people had been getting lactose? The bacteria in the colon adapt to the lactose, says Savaiano, fermenting less of it, and therefore generating fewer and milder symptoms. So, if you consume dairy products regularly, you're less likely to suffer the symptoms of lactose intolerance.

Eat Small Amounts

Another key to symptom-free consumption of dairy foods is to never consume too much dairy at one time. In a study conducted by Savaiano and researchers at the Department of Food Science and Nutrition at the University of Minnesota at St. Paul, published in the *Journal of the American Dietetic Association,* 13 people with lactose intolerance were given challenge doses of the sugar. They received either 2, 6, 12, or 20 grams of lactose in water. For comparison, an 8-ounce cup of milk has about 12 grams of lactose; 8 ounces of yogurt about 10 grams; a scoop of ice cream about 1.5 grams; and 1 ounce of hard, aged cheese, such as cheddar or Swiss, contains almost no lactose. Hydrogen production didn't start going up until the 6-gram dose, abdominal pain didn't begin until 12 grams, and gas didn't begin until 20 grams.

A paper reviewing the current research on lactose intolerance written by scientists at the Foundation for Nutrition Research in Helsinki, Finland, and published in the *Journal of the American College of Nutrition,* says that about one-third to one-half of people with lactose intolerance will experience some symptoms when drinking an 8-ounce cup of milk. So, to be on the safe side, those with lactose intolerance will want to limit their milk intake to no more than 8 ounces at any one time. But there are many strategies to reduce symptoms from milk and there are many types of dairy foods other than milk that are easily digested by people with lactose intolerance.

Eat Dairy with Meals

In some of the studies I've already reported in which people with lactose intolerance didn't have symptoms when they consumed dairy, the dairy was given with a meal. In one study conducted by researchers at the University of Minnesota, published in the *American Journal of Clinical Nutrition,* when 12 people with lactose intolerance had their milk with breakfast, the production of hydrogen was delayed by 4 hours, compared to when they drank milk without a meal. Additionally, only 3 of the 12 study participants had digestive upset when they consumed milk with a meal, compared to 9 who had symptoms when they drank milk by itself. And the severity of the symptoms was reduced when the participants drank milk with a meal, as compared to drinking it alone.

The researchers of this study concluded that people with lactose intolerance "should consume food simultaneously with lactose-containing beverages to reduce intolerance symptoms." Eating dairy with a meal helps because food slows the rate at which lactose leaves your stomach and arrives in the colon, giving whatever lactase is present more time to break down the sugar.

This advice to have dairy with a meal, however, doesn't pertain to midmorning or midafternoon snacks of yogurt or hard cheese. Let's take a look at those two dairy foods.

Eat Yogurt with "Live Cultures"

There are two reasons that yogurt is such a good choice for those with lactose intolerance. Yogurt is part fluid, part solid. The more solid or foodlike the dairy product, the slower it leaves the stomach and the slower it moves through the intestines; thus, the more opportunity lactase has to digest it. As you now know, it's best to consume dairy with food; yogurt is one part food, one part beverage.

Yogurt is a fermented food. Friendly bacteria or live cultures—typically either *Lactobacillus bulgaricus* or *Streptococcus thermophilus*—turn milk into yogurt. These bacteria contain an enzyme that releases lactase, and lactase digests lactose.

In one study published in the *New England Journal of Medicine,* lactose-intolerant people who ate yogurt generated only one-third the amount of hydrogen as those who got the same amount of lactose in milk or added to water. Those who ate the yogurt also experienced much less gas.

In a study on children conducted by researchers in the Department of Pediatrics at the Johns Hopkins University School of Medicine, published in the *American Journal of Clinical Nutrition,* lactose-intolerant kids who ate yogurt containing active cultures had significantly fewer symptoms than children who drank milk.

When choosing a yogurt, look for a product that has the words *live cultures* on the ingredient list. Also, the National Yogurt Association puts a Live and Active Cultures seal on products that contain significant amounts of *Lactobacillus bulgaricus* or *Streptococcus thermophilus.* The program is voluntary for manufacturers, so not every yogurt with live cultures has the seal; but those that do have the seal definitely contain live cultures.

Eat Low-Lactose Hard Cheeses

Hard, aged cheeses like cheddar and Swiss contain minuscule amounts of lactose. If you have lactose intolerance, hard cheeses are a wise choice for at least 1 one of your daily servings of dairy.

Drink Lactose-Reduced or Lactose-Free Milk or Use a Lactase Dietary Aid

Other solutions to the problem of lactose intolerance are to consume dairy *without* lactose or to take a supplement of lactase right before or with dairy. Yes, there are milks that have either low or no levels of lactose. To make these milks, manufacturers add lactase to pasteurized milk, store it for a day or so until the lactose is reduced, then pasteurize it again to stop the process. You can find milk that is lactose-reduced (about 70% of its lactose is removed) or lactose-free (99.99% of its lactose is removed) at most supermarkets. Like regular milk, there are 2%, 1%, and nonfat varieties. These milks typically taste sweeter than regular milks.

You can also find lactase supplements that you can either add to milk or take right before consuming dairy. Scientific studies show that lactose-reduced or lactose-free milk and lactose supplements are very effective in reducing the symptoms of lactose intolerance.

Drink Milk Containing Lactobacillus Acidophilus

Like yogurt, this type of milk contains one or more live, lactose-digesting cultures *(Lactobacillus acidophilus, Streptococcus thermophilus, Lactobacillus bulgaricus,* and *Bifidobacterium bifidus),* but the milk hasn't gone through the fermentation process that produces yogurt.

One caveat is that studies show that acidophilus or other culture-containing milk is nowhere near as effective as yogurt in eliminating or reducing the symptoms of lactose intolerance. But if you have lactose intolerance, you may want to make this type of product part of your dairy intake. In the supermarket, the product is usually called sweet acidophilus milk; it doesn't have the somewhat sour, yogurtlike taste that would occur if the live culture were fermenting the milk.

Try Chocolate Milk

As long as chocolate milk fits into the weight-loss calorie level you've chosen, it's a great way to get dairy and two studies show it may help you avoid the symptoms of lactose intolerance.

4
Week-by-Week
Weight-Loss Success:
The Calcium Key Meal Plans

THE MEAL PLANS in this chapter guide you to a day's eating that is 500 calories below your maintenance level. Obviously, cutting those calories will help you shed pounds. But because the meal plans cut calories and include 3 to 4 servings of dairy a day, you can lose up to 70% more weight and 64% more fat (particularly from around your belly) than you would by just cutting calories.

How to Use the Calcium Key Meal Plans

Before you shop, check out the boldface items in the plans. These items are High-Dairy Recipes that are featured in chapter 5. Add their ingredients to your shopping list. The meal plans are organized week by week. Before each week, review the plans and make a shopping list. Stock up on all the foods you'll need for that week.

Most of the foods in the Free exchange category are either no- or low-calorie; you can add them to the meal plan even if they're not listed. For instance, feel free to dip raw vegetables in fat-free dressing, which is on the Free Foods list on pages 92–93. It also includes lots of spices and condiments, which you can use to add flavor to your meals. When the meal plan says "beverage of choice," it means any free low-calorie beverage, like water, sugar-free sodas, and black coffee, not alcoholic beverages or coffee drinks.

Now that you understand the Calcium Key Exchange System, go ahead and substitute within any exchange category. For example, exchange skim milk for a cup of yogurt, both of which are 1 dairy exchange; or exchange a peach for a cup of raspberries, both of which are 1 fruit exchange. CKES provides a lot of room for personal choice within the meal plans.

Consult the meal plans for holidays and restaurant eating. You'll find meal plans for two holiday meals: one featuring turkey, one featuring beef. You'll also find plans for eating a fast-food burger meal, fast-food chicken meal, sandwich/deli meal, American breakfast meal (at a Perkins, Denny's, Applebee's, or similar establishment), and for dining out on Mexican and Chinese food. The holiday and restaurant meal plans aren't meant as prescriptions. Rather, they're included to give you ideas about the type of holiday and restaurant meals you can eat while staying on CKES.

Use the meal plans only when you want. Maybe you don't like the idea of eating according to a set plan. But maybe there are some days when not having to think about what you're going to eat is helpful. Use a meal plan on that day. It's okay if you don't stay on the meal plans for 5 weeks or even for 1 week. Use them as they fit your inclination and schedule. Of course, that doesn't mean not staying on CKES—that's the overall plan, whether you use the meal plans or not as your guideline.

1200-Calorie Calcium Key Meal Plans

DAY 1

Breakfast
Baked French Toast with Maple Yogurt and Fruit
beverage of choice

Lunch
1½ oz. roasted chicken
½ small baked potato
2 t. butter
1 c. melon balls
1 c. mixed vegetables
1 c. skim milk

Dinner
1 sl. cheese pizza
1 c. raw vegetables
beverage of choice

Snack
½ c. sugar-free pudding

DAY 2

Breakfast
¾ c. cold cereal (unsweetened)
½ c. skim milk
beverage of choice

Lunch
1 pc. string cheese
6 whole-wheat crackers
Fresh Fruit Kebob with Citrus Poppy-Seed Dressing
1 c. raw broccoli/cauliflower
beverage of choice

Dinner
Turkey Tet-rotini
1 c. cooked carrots
lettuce salad
2 T. low-fat salad dressing
½ c. strawberries
beverage of choice

Snack
½ orange

DAY 3

Breakfast
1 sl. whole-wheat toast
1 t. butter
½ c. orange juice
additional beverage of choice

Lunch
½ serving **Tuna Cheese Salad**
vegetable salad
2 T. low-fat salad dressing
beverage of choice

Dinner
⅔ c. **Mediterranean Lentil Soup**
1 c. raw vegetables
2 T. low-fat ranch dressing
1 c. skim milk

Snack
Berry Blue Smoothie

DAY 4

Breakfast
½ c. oatmeal
½ c. skim milk
1 tangerine
beverage of choice

Lunch
cheeseburger (2 oz. meat, 1 sl.
    cheese, ½ bun, lettuce, tomato,
    onion)
1 T. low-fat mayonnaise
Potato Salad
1 watermelon wedge
beverage of choice

Dinner
Eggplant Lasagna
vegetable salad
2 T. low-fat salad dressing
beverage of choice

Snack
½ c. flavored fat-free yogurt
1 small apple

DAY 5

Breakfast
½ bagel
1 T. cream cheese
beverage of choice

Lunch
Pita Shrimp
1½ c. raw vegetables
3 T. low-fat ranch dressing
1 c. skim milk
additional beverage of choice

Dinner
1 oz. roast/grilled pork tenderloin
½ serving **Creamy Spring Risotto**
beverage of choice

Snack
Berry Berry Berry Smoothie

DAY 6

Breakfast
Tammi's Minnesota Muffin
½ grapefruit
½ c. skim milk
additional beverage of choice

Lunch
½ c. low-fat cottage cheese
2 canned peach halves in juice
1 c. vegetable salad
2 T. low-fat salad dressing
beverage of choice

Dinner
**Portabella Mushroom Burger with
    Caramelized Balsamic Onions**
lettuce and tomato slices
1 T. low-fat mayonnaise
½ c. mixed berries
beverage of choice

Snack
Piña Colada Smoothie

DAY 7

Breakfast
¾ c. cold cereal (unsweetened)
1 c. skim milk
1 small banana
beverage of choice

Lunch
Wild Rice Soup
Frozen Fruit Cup
beverage of choice

Dinner
chicken and vegetable stir-fry
(1 oz. chicken, 1 c. vegetables)
⅓ c. cooked brown rice
beverage of choice

Snack
1 apple with 2 t. peanut butter

DAY 8

Breakfast
Sautéed Apple Crepe
1 c. skim milk
additional beverage of choice

Lunch
2 oz. lean baked ham
½ c. cooked asparagus
lettuce salad
2 T. low-fat salad dressing
beverage of choice

Dinner
Tomato Pepper Penne
1 c. raw vegetables
2 T. low-fat ranch dressing
20–25 grapes
beverage of choice

Snack
1 orange

DAY 9

Breakfast
1 English muffin
½ c. fat-free yogurt (artificially
sweetened)
beverage of choice

Lunch
Fruit and Cheese Salad
1 sl. whole-wheat bread
1 c. coleslaw (made with fat-free
dressing)
beverage of choice

Dinner
2 oz. grilled chicken
Tabbouleh Zucchini
lettuce salad
2 T. fat-free salad dressing
beverage of choice

Snack
Cherry Almond Smoothie

DAY 10

Breakfast
¾ c. cold cereal (unsweetened)
½ c. skim milk
beverage of choice

Lunch
Oriental Chicken Salad
3 sl. melba toast
1 t. butter
beverage of choice

Dinner
Chili Cheese Casserole
1 c. cooked broccoli
lettuce salad
2 T. low-fat salad dressing
beverage of choice

Snack
Grape Ape Smoothie

DAY 11

Breakfast
yogurt/fruit parfait (1 c. artificially
sweetened fat-free yogurt and
1 c. berries)
beverage of choice

Lunch
Veggie and Cheese Sub Sandwich
1 tangerine
beverage of choice

Dinner
1 c. beef stew
1 small biscuit
1 t. butter
1 c. sliced cucumber
beverage of choice

Snack
½ c. pudding (artificially sweetened)

DAY 12

Breakfast
½ c. cooked cereal
1 c. skim milk
½ grapefruit
beverage of choice

Lunch
taco with meat and cheese
⅓ c. Spanish rice
1 sliced tomato
beverage of choice

Dinner
½ serving **Parmesan Roughy**
½ c. green beans with 1 T. almonds
½ sl. rye bread
1 t. butter
beverage of choice

Snack
Fuzzy Berry Smoothie

DAY 13

Breakfast
1 frozen waffle

½ c. orange juice
1 T. sugar-free syrup
additional beverage of choice

Lunch
tuna salad sandwich (¼ c. tuna
salad, 1 sl. bread, 1 sl. reduced-
fat cheese, sliced tomato/
romaine lettuce)
1 pear
½ c. skim milk
additional beverage of choice

Dinner
1 oz. grilled beef sirloin
½ c. grilled mushrooms
Stuffed Tomato
¾ c. pineapple
beverage of choice

Snack
1 c. fat-free yogurt (artificially
sweetened)
1½ c. low-fat popcorn

DAY 14

Breakfast
1 c. fat-free yogurt (artificially
sweetened)
½ c. sliced peaches
beverage of choice

Lunch
low-fat hot dog on ½ bun
1 c. raw vegetables
2 T. low-fat ranch dressing
beverage of choice

Dinner
Stuffed Chicken Popover (with
1 oz. chicken)
1 c. zucchini/carrots
Fruit Pizza
beverage of choice

Snack
½ banana with 2 t. peanut butter
½ c. skim milk

DAY 15

Breakfast
Ham and Cheese Muffin
1 orange
1 c. skim milk
additional beverage of choice

Lunch
2 oz. roast turkey
2 T. fat-free gravy
½ serving **Sweet Potato on
the Half Shell**
1 t. butter
1 c. brussels sprouts
beverage of choice

Dinner
1 sl. thin-crust pizza
1 c. vegetable salad
2 T. low-fat salad dressing
beverage of choice

Snack
½ serving **Orange Cream
Smoothie**

DAY 16

Breakfast
¾ c. cold cereal (unsweetened)
1 c. skim milk
beverage of choice

Lunch
½ serving **Greek Couscous Salad**
1 c. raw baby carrots
1 pc. string cheese
beverage of choice

Dinner
½ serving **Pork Stroganoff**
1 c. cooked mixed vegetables
1 c. melon balls
beverage of choice

Snack
Berry Banana Smoothie
18 whole almonds

DAY 17

Breakfast
1 c. yogurt (artificially sweetened)
1 c. raspberries
beverage of choice

Lunch
Cheese Tortellini Soup
1 c. raw vegetables
2 T. low-fat ranch dressing
beverage of choice

Dinner
spaghetti with meat sauce (½ c.
pasta, ½ c. sauce)
1 c. vegetable salad
2 T. low-fat salad dressing
beverage of choice

Snack
½ c. sugar-free pudding

DAY 18

Breakfast
1 sl. raisin toast (unfrosted)
1 t. butter
½ c. apple juice
additional beverage of choice

Lunch
deli plate (1½ oz. reduced-fat
cheese, 1 sliced orange, 1 c.
raw vegetables)
beverage of choice

Dinner
**Chicken Enchilada in White Cream
Sauce**
Mexican Cornbread
1 c. cooked green beans
2 t. butter
beverage of choice

Snack
15 grapes

DAY 19

Breakfast
¾ c. cold cereal
½ c. skim milk
½ grapefruit
beverage of choice

Lunch
½ grilled cheese sandwich
Apple Carrot Salad
1 c. skim milk

Dinner
2 oz. meatloaf
½ c. **Creamy Mashed Potatoes**
2 T. fat-free gravy
1 c. cooked carrots
1 t. butter
beverage of choice

Snack
½ c. frozen vanilla yogurt

DAY 20

Breakfast
½ c. oatmeal
1 c. skim milk
½ c. orange juice
additional beverage of choice

Lunch
large vegetable salad
¼ c. low-fat dressing
1 small roll
1 t. butter
beverage of choice

Dinner
Grilled Fish Taco
beverage of choice

Snack
Cherry Almond Smoothie

DAY 21

Breakfast
½ English muffin
1 c. berries
1 t. butter
beverage of choice

Lunch
Baked Potato Soup
2 c. raw vegetables
2 T. low-fat ranch dressing
¾ c. pineapple
beverage of choice

Dinner
Pizza Burger with 1 sl. bread
½ c. cooked mixed vegetables
beverage of choice

Snack
½ c. fat-free yogurt (artificially
sweetened)
¾ c. peach slices

DAY 22

Breakfast
½ bagel
2 T. cream cheese
½ c. juice blend
beverage of choice

Lunch
Hashbrown Quiche
Melon Berry Soup
beverage of choice

Dinner
1 oz. barbecued beef on bun
¼ c. baked beans
½ c. raw baby carrots
2 T. low-fat ranch dressing
beverage of choice

Snack
Piña Colada Smoothie

DAY 23

Breakfast
¾ c. cold cereal (unsweetened)
1 c. skim milk
beverage of choice

Lunch
⅔ c. **Chicken Enchilada Soup**
½ c. vegetable salad
2 T. low-fat salad dressing
beverage of choice

Dinner
Creamy Sausage Creole
½ c. cooked green beans with
    1 T. almonds
beverage of choice

Snack
Berry Berry Berry Smoothie

DAY 24

Breakfast
1 c. yogurt (artificially sweetened)
¾ c. blueberries
beverage of choice

Lunch
beef and cheese quesadilla (1½ oz.
    reduced-fat cheese, 1½ oz.
    cooked ground beef, two 6"
    flour tortillas)
1 sliced tomato
2 T. sour cream
salsa
beverage of choice

Dinner
Reuben Pizza
2 c. vegetable salad
2 T. low-fat salad dressing
1 peach
beverage of choice

Snack
1 watermelon wedge

DAY 25

Breakfast
½ English muffin
2 t. butter
beverage of choice

Lunch
**Grilled Turkey, Vegetable, and
    Cheese Sandwich**
½ c. cooked spinach
½ c. tomato/vegetable juice
additional beverage of choice

Dinner
1 oz. baked salmon fillet
¼ c. green peas
1 t. butter
½ c. skim milk
additional beverage of choice

Snack
Tropical Smoothie

DAY 26

Breakfast
½ c. cooked cereal
½ c. skim milk
beverage of choice

Lunch
½ c. chili/beans with 1 oz.
    reduced-fat cheese
1 c. raw vegetables
2 T. low-fat ranch dressing
beverage of choice

Dinner
Stromboli
1 c. cooked broccoli/cauliflower
1 t. butter
beverage of choice

Snack
Creamy Peach Smoothie

DAY 27

Breakfast
¾ c. cold cereal (unsweetened)
½ c. skim milk
1 banana
beverage of choice

Lunch
½ serving **Caesar Tortellini
Salad**
2 T. sunflower seeds
1 orange
beverage of choice

Dinner
1 oz. grilled pork chop
1 c. grilled vegetables
1 c. skim milk

Snack
1 c. sugar-free pudding

DAY 28

Breakfast
yogurt/fruit parfait (½ c. artificially
sweetened fat-free yogurt and
1 c. berries)
3 T. Grape Nuts cereal (sprinkled
over parfait)
beverage of choice

Lunch
Chef's Pasta Salad
1 c. melon balls
1 c. tomato/vegetable juice
additional beverage of
choice

Dinner
Fajita Lettuce Wrap (with
1 oz. beef)
2 T. sour cream
beverage of choice

Snack
1 pear
12 almonds

1400-Calorie Calcium Key Meal Plans

DAY 1

Breakfast
**Baked French Toast with Maple
Yogurt and Fruit**
beverage of choice

Lunch
2½ oz. roasted chicken
½ small baked potato
1 t. butter
1 c. melon balls
1 c. mixed vegetables
1 c. skim milk

Dinner
1 sl. cheese pizza
1 c. raw vegetables
1½ c. pineapple
beverage of choice

Snack
½ c. sugar-free pudding

DAY 2

Breakfast
 ¾ c. cold cereal (unsweetened)
 ½ c. skim milk
 ½ c. orange juice
 1 hard-cooked egg
 beverage of choice

Lunch
 1 pc. string cheese
 6 whole-wheat crackers
 **Fresh Fruit Kebob with Citrus
  Poppy-Seed Dressing**
 1 c. raw broccoli/cauliflower
 beverage of choice

Dinner
 Turkey Tet-rotini
 1 c. cooked carrots
 lettuce salad
 2 T. low-fat salad dressing
 1 c. strawberries
 beverage of choice

Snack
 1 orange

DAY 3

Breakfast
 1 sl. whole-wheat toast
 1 t. butter
 ½ c. orange juice
 additional beverage of choice

Lunch
 Tuna Cheese Salad
 vegetable salad
 2 T. low-fat salad dressing
 1 peach
 beverage of choice

Dinner
 ⅔ c. **Mediterranean Lentil Soup**
 1 c. raw vegetables
 2 T. fat-free ranch dressing
 1 c. skim milk

Snack
 Berry Blue Smoothie

DAY 4

Breakfast
 ½ c. oatmeal
 ½ c. skim milk
 1 tangerine
 beverage of choice

Lunch
 cheeseburger (3 oz. meat, 1 sl.
  cheese, 1 bun, lettuce, tomato,
  onion)
 1 T. low-fat mayonnaise
 Potato Salad
 1 watermelon wedge
 beverage of choice

Dinner
 Eggplant Lasagna
 vegetable salad
 2 T. low-fat salad dressing
 ½ c. fruit salad
 beverage of choice

Snack
 ½ c. flavored fat-free yogurt
 1 small apple

DAY 5

Breakfast
 ½ bagel
 1 T. cream cheese
 ½ c. orange juice
 additional beverage of choice

Lunch
 Pita Shrimp
 lettuce salad
 1 T. low-fat salad dressing
 1 plum
 beverage of choice

Dinner
 2 oz. roast/grilled pork
  tenderloin
 Creamy Spring Risotto
 beverage of choice

Snack
 Berry Berry Berry Smoothie

DAY 6

Breakfast
Tammi's Minnesota Muffin
½ grapefruit
½ c. skim milk
additional beverage of choice

Lunch
½ c. low-fat cottage cheese
2 canned peach halves in juice
1 oz. deli lean ham/turkey
1 c. vegetable salad
2 T. fat-free salad dressing
1 soft bread stick
beverage of choice

Dinner
Portabella Mushroom Burger with Caramelized Balsamic Onions
lettuce and tomato slices
1 T. low-fat mayonnaise
1½ c. mixed berries
beverage of choice

Snack
Piña Colada Smoothie

DAY 7

Breakfast
¾ c. cold cereal (unsweetened)
1 c. skim milk
1 small banana
beverage of choice

Lunch
Wild Rice Soup
6 whole-wheat crackers
Frozen Fruit Cup
beverage of choice

Dinner
chicken and vegetable stir-fry
(2 oz. chicken, 1 c. vegetables)
⅓ c. cooked brown rice
⅛ honeydew melon
beverage of choice

Snack
1 apple with 2 t. peanut butter

DAY 8

Breakfast
2 **Sautéed Apple Crepes**
1 c. skim milk
additional beverage of choice

Lunch
3 oz. lean baked ham
½ c. cooked asparagus
lettuce salad
2 T. low-fat salad dressing
¾ c. peach slices
beverage of choice

Dinner
Tomato Pepper Penne
1 c. raw vegetables
2 T. low-fat ranch dressing
15 grapes
beverage of choice

Snack
1 orange

DAY 9

Breakfast
1 English muffin
½ c. fat-free yogurt (artificially
sweetened)
½ banana
beverage of choice

Lunch
Fruit and Cheese Salad
1 sl. whole-wheat bread
1 c. coleslaw (made with fat-free
dressing)
beverage of choice

Dinner
3 oz. grilled chicken
Tabbouleh Zucchini
½ c. corn
lettuce salad
2 T. fat-free salad dressing
beverage of choice

Snack
Cherry Almond Smoothie

DAY 10

Breakfast
1 c. cold cereal (unsweetened)
½ c. skim milk
beverage of choice

Lunch
Oriental Chicken Salad
6 sl. melba toast
1 t. butter
beverage of choice

Dinner
Chili Cheese Casserole
1 c. cooked broccoli
lettuce salad
2 T. low-fat salad dressing
1 watermelon wedge
beverage of choice

Snack
Grape Ape Smoothie

DAY 11

Breakfast
yogurt/fruit parfait (1 c. artificially
    sweetened fat-free yogurt and
    1 c. berries)
beverage of choice

Lunch
Veggie and Cheese Sub Sandwich
2 tangerines
beverage of choice

Dinner
1½ c. beef stew
1 small biscuit
1 c. sliced cucumber
½ c. canned fruit (unsweetened)
beverage of choice

Snack
½ c. pudding (artificially
    sweetened)

DAY 12

Breakfast
1 c. cooked cereal
½ c. skim milk
½ grapefruit
beverage of choice

Lunch
taco with meat and cheese
⅓ c. Spanish rice
1 sliced tomato
½ c. unsweetened applesauce
beverage of choice

Dinner
Parmesan Roughy
½ c. green beans
½ sl. rye bread
1 t. butter
beverage of choice

Snack
Fuzzy Berry Smoothie

DAY 13

Breakfast
1 frozen waffle
1 c. orange juice
1 T. sugar-free syrup
additional beverage of choice

Lunch
tuna salad sandwich (¼ c. tuna
    salad, 2 sl. bread, 1 sl. reduced-
    fat cheese, sliced tomato/
    romaine lettuce)
1 pear
½ c. skim milk
additional beverage of choice

Dinner
2 oz. grilled beef sirloin
½ c. grilled mushrooms
Stuffed Tomato
¾ c. pineapple
beverage of choice

Snack
1 c. fat-free yogurt (artificially
    sweetened)
1½ c. low-fat popcorn

DAY 14

Breakfast
1 c. fat-free yogurt (artificially
  sweetened)
½ c. sliced peaches
beverage of choice

Lunch
low-fat hot dog on bun
1 c. raw vegetables
2 T. fat-free ranch dressing
beverage of choice

Dinner
Stuffed Chicken Popover
1 c. zucchini/carrots
Fruit Pizza
beverage of choice

Snack
1 banana with 2 t. peanut butter
½ c. skim milk

DAY 15

Breakfast
Ham and Cheese Muffin
1 orange
1 c. skim milk
additional beverage of choice

Lunch
3 oz. roast turkey
2 T. fat-free gravy
Sweet Potato on the Half Shell
1 t. butter
1 c. brussels sprouts
½ small dinner roll
beverage of choice

Dinner
1 sl. thin-crust pizza
1 c. vegetable salad
2 T. fat-free salad dressing
1 plum
beverage of choice

Snack
½ serving **Orange Cream Smoothie**

DAY 16

Breakfast
¾ c. cold cereal (unsweetened)
1 c. skim milk
½ c. orange or apple juice
additional beverage of choice

Lunch
½ serving **Greek Couscous
  Salad**
1 c. raw baby carrots
1 pc. string cheese
beverage of choice

Dinner
Pork Stroganoff
1 c. cooked mixed vegetables
1 c. melon balls
beverage of choice

Snack
Berry Banana Smoothie
12 whole almonds

DAY 17

Breakfast
1 c. fat-free yogurt (artificially
  sweetened)
1 c. raspberries
1 scrambled egg
beverage of choice

Lunch
Cheese Tortellini Soup
1 c. raw vegetables
2 T. low-fat ranch dressing
24 oyster crackers
beverage of choice

Dinner
spaghetti with meat sauce
  (½ c. pasta, ½ c. sauce)
1 c. vegetable salad
2 T. low-fat salad dressing
1 small apple
beverage of choice

Snack
½ c. sugar-free pudding

DAY 18

Breakfast
1 sl. raisin toast (unfrosted)
1 t. butter
½ c. apple juice
additional beverage of choice

Lunch
deli plate (1 oz. lean deli meat,
    1½ oz. reduced-fat cheese,
    1 sliced orange, 1 c. raw
    vegetables)
1 small whole-wheat roll
beverage of choice

Dinner
**Chicken Enchilada in White Cream
    Sauce**
Mexican Cornbread
1 c. cooked green beans
1 t. butter
½ c. fruit salad
beverage of choice

Snack
15 grapes

DAY 19

Breakfast
¾ c. cold cereal
½ c. skim milk
½ grapefruit
beverage of choice

Lunch
grilled cheese sandwich
Apple Carrot Salad
½ c. skim milk
additional beverage of choice

Dinner
3 oz. meatloaf
½ c. **Creamy Mashed Potatoes**
2 T. fat-free gravy
1 c. cooked carrots
1 nectarine
beverage of choice

Snack
½ c. frozen vanilla yogurt

DAY 20

Breakfast
1 c. oatmeal
1 c. skim milk
½ c. orange juice
beverage of choice

Lunch
large vegetable salad
¼ c. fat-free dressing
¼ c. low-fat cottage cheese
1 small roll
1 t. butter
beverage of choice

Dinner
Grilled Fish Taco
1 c. melon balls
beverage of choice

Snack
Cherry Almond Smoothie

DAY 21

Breakfast
½ English muffin
1 c. berries
1 t. butter
1 poached egg
beverage of choice

Lunch
Baked Potato Soup
2 c. raw vegetables
2 T. fat-free ranch dressing
¾ c. pineapple
beverage of choice

Dinner
Pizza Burger
½ c. cooked mixed vegetables
½ c. canned fruit (unsweetened)
beverage of choice

Snack
½ c. fat-free yogurt (artificially
    sweetened)
¾ c. peach slices

DAY 22

Breakfast
½ bagel
1 T. cream cheese
1 c. juice blend

Lunch
Hashbrown Quiche
Melon Berry Soup
1 c. vegetable salad
2 T. fat-free salad dressing
beverage of choice

Dinner
2 oz. barbecued beef on bun
¼ c. baked beans
1 c. raw baby carrots
2 T. low-fat ranch dressing
beverage of choice

Snack
Piña Colada Smoothie

DAY 23

Breakfast
¾ c. cold cereal (unsweetened)
1 c. skim milk
½ c. orange juice
additional beverage of choice

Lunch
Chicken Enchilada Soup
1 c. lettuce salad
2 T. low-fat salad dressing
beverage of choice

Dinner
Creamy Sausage Creole
½ c. cooked green beans with 1 T.
    almonds
beverage of choice

Snack
Berry Berry Berry Smoothie

DAY 24

Breakfast
1 c. fat-free yogurt (artificially
    sweetened)
¾ c. blueberries
¼ c. fat-free granola
beverage of choice

Lunch
beef and cheese quesadilla (1½ oz.
    reduced-fat cheese, 2½ oz.
    cooked ground beef, two 6" flour
    tortillas)
1 sliced tomato
2 T. sour cream
salsa
beverage of choice

Dinner
Reuben Pizza
2 c. vegetable salad
2 T. low-fat salad dressing
1 peach
beverage of choice

Snack
2 watermelon wedges

DAY 25

Breakfast
1 English muffin
2 t. butter
beverage of choice

Lunch
Grilled Turkey, Vegetable, and
    Cheese Sandwich
½ c. cooked spinach
½ c. tomato/vegetable juice
beverage of choice

Dinner
2 oz. baked salmon fillet
¼ c. green peas
½ c. skim milk
½ c. applesauce (unsweetened)
additional beverage of choice

Snack
Tropical Smoothie

DAY 26

Breakfast
½ c. cooked cereal
½ c. skim milk
beverage of choice

Lunch
1 c. chili/beans with 1 oz.
  reduced-fat cheese
1 c. raw vegetables
2 T. fat-free ranch dressing
beverage of choice

Dinner
Stromboli
1 c. cooked broccoli/cauliflower
1 c. mixed berries
beverage of choice

Snack
Creamy Peach Smoothie

DAY 27

Breakfast
¾ c. cold cereal (unsweetened)
1 c. skim milk
1 banana
beverage of choice

Lunch
Caesar Tortellini Salad
¼ c. low-fat croutons
1 T. sunflower seeds
1 orange
beverage of choice

Dinner
1 oz. grilled pork chop
1 c. grilled vegetables
1 baked apple
beverage of choice

Snack
1 c. sugar-free pudding

DAY 28

Breakfast
yogurt/fruit parfait (½ c. artificially
  sweetened fat-free yogurt and
  1 c. berries)
3 T. Grape Nuts cereal (sprinkled
  over parfait)
beverage of choice

Lunch
Chef's Pasta Salad
1 c. melon balls
1 c. tomato/vegetable juice
additional beverage of choice

Dinner
Fajita Lettuce Wrap
2 T. sour cream
½ c. canned fruit (unsweetened)
½ large ear corn on the cob
1 t. butter
beverage of choice

Snack
1 pear

1600-Calorie Calcium Key Meal Plans

DAY 1

Breakfast
**Baked French Toast with Maple
  Yogurt and Fruit**
beverage of choice

Lunch
3½ oz. roasted chicken
1 medium baked potato
1 t. butter
1 c. melon balls
1 c. mixed vegetables

1 c. skim milk
additional beverage of choice

Dinner
1 sl. cheese pizza
1 c. raw vegetables
1½ c. pineapple
beverage of choice

Snack
½ c. sugar-free pudding

DAY 2

Breakfast
¾ c. cold cereal (unsweetened)
½ c. skim milk
½ c. orange juice
1 hard-cooked egg
beverage of choice

Lunch
1 pc. string cheese
6 whole-wheat crackers
**Fresh Fruit Kebob with Citrus
Poppy-Seed Dressing**
1 c. raw broccoli/cauliflower
beverage of choice

Dinner
Turkey Tet-rotini
1 c. cooked carrots
lettuce salad
2 T. low-fat salad dressing
1 c. strawberries
beverage of choice

Snack
1 oz. turkey
1 sl. whole-wheat bread
1 orange

DAY 3

Breakfast
1 sl. whole-wheat toast
1 t. butter
½ c. orange juice

additional beverage of choice

Lunch
Tuna Cheese Salad
vegetable salad
2 T. low-fat salad dressing
1 peach
beverage of choice

Dinner
Mediterranean Lentil Soup
1 c. raw vegetables
2 T. fat-free ranch dressing
3 whole-wheat crackers
beverage of choice

Snack
Berry Blue Smoothie

DAY 4

Breakfast
½ c. oatmeal
½ c. skim milk
1 tangerine
beverage of choice

Lunch
cheeseburger (4 oz. meat, 1 sl.
cheese, 1 bun, lettuce, tomato,
onion)
1 T. low-fat mayonnaise
Potato Salad
1 watermelon wedge
beverage of choice

Dinner
Eggplant Lasagna
vegetable salad
2 T. low-fat salad dressing
½ c. fruit salad
1 sl. French bread
1 t. butter
beverage of choice

Snack
½ c. flavored fat-free yogurt
1 small apple

DAY 5

Breakfast
½ bagel
1 T. cream cheese
½ c. orange juice
beverage of choice

Lunch
Pita Shrimp
lettuce salad
1 T. low-fat dressing
1 plum
beverage of choice

Dinner
3 oz. roast/grilled pork tenderloin
Creamy Spring Risotto
1 sl. bread
beverage of choice

Snack
Berry Berry Berry Smoothie

DAY 6

Breakfast
Tammi's Minnesota Muffin
½ grapefruit
½ c. skim milk
additional beverage of choice

Lunch
½ c. low-fat cottage cheese
2 canned peach halves in juice
2 oz. deli lean ham/turkey
1 c. vegetable salad
2 T. fat-free salad dressing
2 soft bread sticks
beverage of choice

Dinner
**Portabella Mushroom Burger with
    Caramelized Balsamic Onions**
lettuce and tomato slices
1 T. low-fat mayonnaise
1½ c. mixed berries
beverage of choice

Snack
Piña Colada Smoothie

DAY 7

Breakfast
¾ c. cold cereal (unsweetened)
1 c. skim milk
1 small banana
beverage of choice

Lunch
Wild Rice Soup
6 whole-wheat crackers
Frozen Fruit Cup
beverage of choice

Dinner
chicken and vegetable stir-fry (3 oz.
    chicken, 1 c. vegetables)
⅔ c. cooked brown rice
⅛ honeydew melon
beverage of choice

Snack
1 apple with 2 t. peanut butter

DAY 8

Breakfast
2 Sautéed Apple Crepes
1 c. skim milk
additional beverage of choice

Lunch
4 oz. lean baked ham
½ c. cooked asparagus
lettuce salad
2 T. low-fat salad dressing
¾ c. peach slices
1 small dinner roll
beverage of choice

Dinner
Tomato Pepper Penne
1 c. raw vegetables
2 T. low-fat ranch dressing
15 grapes
beverage of choice

Snack
1 orange

DAY 9

Breakfast
1 English muffin
½ c. fat-free yogurt (artificially
    sweetened)
½ banana
beverage of choice

Lunch
Fruit and Cheese Salad
1 sl. whole-wheat bread
1 c. coleslaw (made with fat-free
    dressing)
beverage of choice

Dinner
4 oz. grilled chicken
Tabbouleh Zucchini
1 c. corn
lettuce salad
2 T. fat-free salad dressing
beverage of choice

Snack
Cherry Almond Smoothie

DAY 10

Breakfast
1 c. cold cereal (unsweetened)
½ c. skim milk
hard-cooked egg
beverage of choice

Lunch
Oriental Chicken Salad
6 sl. melba toast
1 t. butter
beverage of choice

Dinner
Chili Cheese Casserole
1 c. cooked broccoli
lettuce salad
2 T. low-fat salad dressing
1 watermelon wedge
beverage of choice

Snack
Grape Ape Smoothie
1 fat-free granola bar

DAY 11

Breakfast
yogurt/fruit parfait (1 c. artificially
    sweetened fat-free yogurt and
    1 c. berries)
beverage of choice

Lunch
Veggie and Cheese Sub Sandwich
2 tangerines
beverage of choice

Dinner
2 c. beef stew
1 small biscuit
1 c. sliced cucumber
½ c. canned fruit (unsweetened)
beverage of choice

Snack
½ c. pudding (artificially
    sweetened)

DAY 12

Breakfast
1 c. cooked cereal
1 c. skim milk
½ grapefruit
beverage of choice

Lunch
taco with meat and cheese
⅓ c. Spanish rice
1 sliced tomato
½ c. unsweetened applesauce
beverage of choice

Dinner
Parmesan Roughy
½ c. green beans with 1 T.
    almonds
1½ sl. rye bread
1 t. butter
beverage of choice

Snack
Fuzzy Berry Smoothie

DAY 13

Breakfast
1 frozen waffle
1 c. orange juice
1 T. sugar-free syrup
additional beverage of choice

Lunch
tuna salad sandwich (¼ c. tuna
    salad, 2 sl. bread, 1 sl.
    reduced-fat cheese, sliced
    tomato/romaine lettuce)
1 pear
½ c. skim milk
additional beverage of choice

Dinner
3 oz. grilled beef sirloin
½ c. grilled mushrooms
Stuffed Tomato
¾ c. pineapple
1 small dinner roll

Snack
1 c. fat-free yogurt (artificially
    sweetened)
1½ c. low-fat popcorn

DAY 14

Breakfast
1 c. fat-free yogurt (artificially
    sweetened)
½ c. sliced peaches
½ bagel
1 T. reduced-fat cream cheese
beverage of choice

Lunch
low-fat hot dog on bun
1 c. raw vegetables
2 T. fat-free ranch dressing
¼ c. low-fat cottage cheese
beverage of choice

Dinner
Stuffed Chicken Popovers
1 c. zucchini/carrots
Fruit Pizza
beverage of choice

Snack
1 banana with 2 t. peanut butter
½ c. skim milk

DAY 15

Breakfast
Ham and Cheese Muffin
1 orange
½ c. skim milk
additional beverage of choice

Lunch
4 oz. roast turkey
2 T. fat-free gravy
Sweet Potato on the Half Shell
1 c. brussels sprouts
½ dinner roll
beverage of choice

Dinner
2 sl. thin-crust pizza
1 c. vegetable salad
2 T. fat-free salad dressing
1 plum
beverage of choice

Snack
½ serving **Orange Cream Smoothie**

DAY 16

Breakfast
¾ c. cold cereal (unsweetened)
1 c. skim milk
½ c. orange or apple juice

Lunch
Greek Couscous Salad
1 c. raw baby carrots
1 pc. string cheese
beverage of choice

Dinner
Pork Stroganoff
1 c. cooked mixed vegetables
1 c. melon balls
beverage of choice

Snack
Berry Banana Smoothie
12 whole almonds

DAY 17

Breakfast
1 c. fat-free yogurt (artificially
   sweetened)
1 c. raspberries
1 scrambled egg
beverage of choice

Lunch
Cheese Tortellini Soup
1 c. raw vegetables
2 T. low-fat ranch dressing
12 oyster crackers
beverage of choice

Dinner
spaghetti with meat sauce
   (¾ c. pasta, 1 c. sauce)
1 c. lettuce salad
2 T. low-fat salad dressing
1 small apple
beverage of choice

Snack
1 c. sugar-free pudding

DAY 18

Breakfast
2 sl. raisin toast (unfrosted)
1 t. butter
½ c. apple juice
beverage of choice

Lunch
deli plate (2 oz. lean deli meat, 1½
   oz. reduced-fat cheese, 1 sliced
   orange, 1 c. raw vegetables)
1 small whole-wheat roll
beverage of choice

Dinner
**Chicken Enchilada in White Cream
   Sauce**
Mexican Cornbread
1 c. cooked green beans
1 t. butter
½ c. fruit salad
beverage of choice

Snack
15 grapes

DAY 19

Breakfast
¾ c. cold cereal
½ c. skim milk
½ grapefruit
beverage of choice

Lunch
grilled cheese sandwich
Apple Carrot Salad
beverage of choice

Dinner
4 oz. meatloaf
Creamy Mashed Potatoes
2 T. fat-free gravy
1 c. cooked carrots
1 nectarine
beverage of choice

Snack
½ c. frozen vanilla yogurt

DAY 20

Breakfast
1 c. oatmeal
1 c. skim milk
½ c. orange juice
additional beverage of choice

Lunch
large vegetable salad
¼ c. fat-free dressing
1 small roll
1 t. butter
beverage of choice

Dinner
2 Grilled Fish Tacos
beverage of choice

Snack
Cherry Almond Smoothie

DAY 21

Breakfast
1 English muffin
1 c. berries
1 t. butter
1 poached egg
beverage of choice

Lunch
Baked Potato Soup
2 c. raw vegetables
2 T. fat-free ranch dressing
¾ c. pineapple
beverage of choice

Dinner
Pizza Burger
½ c. cooked mixed vegetables
½ c. canned fruit
  (unsweetened)
¼ c. low-fat cottage cheese
beverage of choice

Snack
½ c. fat-free yogurt (artificially
  sweetened)
¾ c. peach slices

DAY 22

Breakfast
½ bagel
1 T. cream cheese
1 c. juice blend
additional beverage of choice

Lunch
Hashbrown Quiche
Melon Berry Soup
1 c. vegetable salad
2 T. fat-free salad dressing
beverage of choice

Dinner
3 oz. barbecued beef on bun
½ c. baked beans
1 c. raw baby carrots

2 T. low-fat ranch dressing
beverage of choice

Snack
Piña Colada Smoothie

DAY 23

Breakfast
¾ c. cold cereal (unsweetened)
1 c. skim milk
½ c. orange juice
additional beverage of choice

Lunch
Chicken Enchilada Soup
1 c. lettuce salad
2 T. low-fat salad dressing
¼ c. low-fat cottage cheese
½ c. fruit cocktail
  (unsweetened)
beverage of choice

Dinner
Creamy Sausage Creole
½ c. cooked green beans with 1 T.
  almonds
beverage of choice

Snack
Berry Berry Berry Smoothie

DAY 24

Breakfast
1 c. fat-free yogurt (artificially
  sweetened)
¾ c. blueberries
¼ c. fat-free granola
beverage of choice

Lunch
beef and cheese quesadilla (1½ oz.
  reduced-fat cheese, 2½ oz.
  cooked ground beef, two 6" flour
  tortillas)

1 sliced tomato
2 T. fat-free sour cream
salsa
beverage of choice

Dinner
Reuben Pizza
2 c. vegetable salad
2 T. fat-free salad dressing
1 peach
beverage of choice

Snack
2 watermelon wedges
1 sl. of bread with 2 T. peanut
    butter

DAY 25

Breakfast
1 English muffin
2 t. butter
beverage of choice

Lunch
**Grilled Turkey, Vegetable, and
    Cheese Sandwich**
½ c. cooked spinach
½ c. tomato/vegetable juice
beverage of choice

Dinner
3 oz. baked salmon fillet
½ c. green peas
½ c. cooked carrots
½ c. skim milk
½ c. applesauce
    (unsweetened)
additional beverage of choice

Snack
Tropical Smoothie

DAY 26

Breakfast
½ c. cooked cereal
½ c. skim milk
½ c. orange juice
additional beverage of choice

Lunch
1 c. chili/beans with 2 oz.
    reduced-fat cheese
1 c. raw vegetables
2 T. fat-free ranch dressing
beverage of choice

Dinner
Stromboli
1 c. cooked broccoli/cauliflower
1 c. mixed berries
beverage of choice

Snack
Creamy Peach Smoothie

DAY 27

Breakfast
¾ c. cold cereal (unsweetened)
1 c. skim milk
1 banana
beverage of choice

Lunch
Caesar Tortellini Salad
¼ c. low-fat croutons
1 T. sunflower seeds
1 orange
beverage of choice

Dinner
2 oz. grilled pork chop
1 c. grilled vegetables
1 baked apple
1 small dinner roll
beverage of choice

Snack
1 c. sugar-free pudding

DAY 28

Breakfast
yogurt/fruit parfait (1/2 c. artificially
    sweetened nonfat yogurt and
    1 c. berries)
3 T. Grape Nuts cereal (sprinkled
    over parfait)
beverage of choice

Lunch
Chef's Pasta Salad
1 c. melon balls

1 c. tomato/vegetable juice
additional beverage of choice

Dinner
Fajita Lettuce Wrap
2 T. fat-free sour cream
1/2 c. canned fruit (unsweetened)
1/2 large ear corn on the cob
beverage of choice

Snack
1 sl. bread with 2 T. peanut butter
1 pear

1800-Calorie Calcium Key Meal Plans

DAY 1

Breakfast
**Baked French Toast with Maple
    Yogurt and Fruit**
beverage of choice

Lunch
3 1/2 oz. roasted chicken
1 medium baked potato
2 T. fat-free sour cream
1 c. melon balls
1 c. mixed vegetables
1 c. skim milk
additional beverage of choice

Dinner
2 sl. cheese pizza
1 c. raw vegetables
1 1/2 c. pineapple
beverage of choice

Snack
1/2 c. sugar-free pudding

DAY 2

Breakfast
3/4 c. cold cereal (unsweetened)
1/2 c. skim milk
1/2 c. orange juice
1 hard-cooked egg
1 sl. whole-wheat toast
1 t. butter
additional beverage of choice

Lunch
1 pc. string cheese
12 whole-wheat crackers
**Fresh Fruit Kebob with Citrus
    Poppy-Seed Dressing**
1 c. raw broccoli/cauliflower
beverage of choice

Dinner
Turkey Tet-rotini
1 1/2 c. cooked carrots
lettuce salad
2 T. low-fat salad dressing
1 c. strawberries
beverage of choice

Snack
1 oz. turkey
1 sl. whole-wheat bread
1 orange

DAY 3

Breakfast
2 sl. whole-wheat toast
1 t. butter
½ c. orange juice
additional beverage of choice

Lunch
Tuna Cheese Salad
vegetable salad
2 T. low-fat salad dressing
1 peach
½ c. tomato juice
additional beverage of choice

Dinner
Mediterranean Lentil Soup
1 c. raw vegetables
2 T. fat-free ranch dressing
3 whole-wheat crackers
beverage of choice

Snack
Berry Blue Smoothie
3 squares graham crackers

DAY 4

Breakfast
1 c. oatmeal
½ c. skim milk
1 tangerine
beverage of choice

Lunch
cheeseburger (4 oz. meat, 1 sl.
    cheese, 1 bun, lettuce, tomato,
    onion)
1 T. low-fat mayonnaise
Potato Salad
1 c. raw vegetable sticks
1 watermelon wedge
beverage of choice

Dinner
Eggplant Lasagna
vegetable salad
2 T. low-fat salad dressing

½ c. fruit salad
2 sl. French bread
1 t. butter
beverage of choice

Snack
½ c. flavored fat-free yogurt
1 small apple

DAY 5

Breakfast
1 bagel
1 T. cream cheese
½ c. orange juice
additional beverage of choice

Lunch
Pita Shrimp
1 c. raw vegetables
1 T. low-fat dressing
1 plum
beverage of choice

Dinner
3 oz. roast/grilled pork tenderloin
Creamy Spring Risotto
2 sl. bread
beverage of choice

Snack
Berry Berry Berry Smoothie

DAY 6

Breakfast
2 **Tammi's Minnesota Muffins**
½ grapefruit
beverage of choice

Lunch
½ c. low-fat cottage cheese
2 canned peach halves in juice
2 oz. deli lean ham/turkey
1 c. vegetable salad
2 T. fat-free salad dressing
2 soft bread sticks
beverage of choice

Dinner
Portabella Mushroom Burger with Caramelized Balsamic Onions
lettuce and tomato slices
1 T. low-fat mayonnaise
6 spears grilled asparagus
1½ c. berries
beverage of choice

Snack
Piña Colada Smoothie
1 low-fat granola bar

DAY 7

Breakfast
¾ c. cold cereal (unsweetened)
1 c. skim milk
1 small banana
beverage of choice

Lunch
Wild Rice Soup
6 whole-wheat crackers
Frozen Fruit Cup
beverage of choice

Dinner
chicken and vegetable stir-fry
   (3 oz. chicken, 1½ c.
   vegetables)
1 c. cooked brown rice
⅛ honeydew melon
beverage of choice

Snack
1 apple with 2 t. peanut butter
½ c. small pretzel twists

DAY 8

Breakfast
2 Sautéed Apple Crepes
1 c. skim milk
additional beverage of choice

Lunch
4 oz. lean baked ham

1 c. cooked asparagus
lettuce salad
2 T. low-fat salad dressing
¾ c. peach slices
1 small dinner roll
beverage of choice

Dinner
Tomato Pepper Penne
1 c. raw vegetables
2 T. low-fat ranch dressing
15 grapes
1 sl. French bread
beverage of choice

Snack
1 orange
3 squares graham crackers

DAY 9

Breakfast
English muffin
½ c. fat-free yogurt (artificially
   sweetened)
½ banana
beverage of choice

Lunch
Fruit and Cheese Salad
2 sl. whole-wheat bread
1 c. coleslaw (made with fat-free
   dressing)
beverage of choice

Dinner
4 oz. grilled chicken
Tabbouleh Zucchini
1 c. corn
lettuce salad
2 T. fat-free salad dressing
1 sl. whole-wheat bread
beverage of choice

Snack
Cherry Almond Smoothie
1 c. raw baby carrots

DAY 10

Breakfast
1 c. cold cereal (unsweetened)
½ c. skim milk
1 hard-cooked egg
beverage of choice

Lunch
Oriental Chicken Salad
6 sl. melba toast
1 t. butter
8 animal crackers
beverage of choice

Dinner
Chili Cheese Casserole
1 c. cooked broccoli
1 c. vegetable salad
2 T. fat-free salad dressing
2-inch-square cornbread
1 watermelon wedge
beverage of choice

Snack
Grape Ape Smoothie
1 fat-free granola bar

DAY 11

Breakfast
yogurt/fruit parfait (1 c. artificially
    sweetened fat-free yogurt and
    1 c. berries)
3 T. Grape Nuts cereal (sprinkled
    over parfait)
beverage of choice

Lunch
Veggie and Cheese Sub Sandwich
2 tangerines
beverage of choice

Dinner
2 c. beef stew
1 small biscuit
1 c. sliced cucumber
½ c. canned fruit (unsweetened)
beverage of choice

Snack
1 c. pudding (artificially sweetened)

DAY 12

Breakfast
1 c. cooked cereal
1 c. skim milk
½ grapefruit
beverage of choice

Lunch
taco with meat and cheese
⅔ c. Spanish rice
1 sliced tomato
½ c. unsweetened applesauce
beverage of choice

Dinner
Parmesan Roughy
1 c. green beans with 2 T.
    almonds
2 sl. rye bread
1 t. butter
beverage of choice

Snack
Fuzzy Berry Smoothie
3 vanilla wafers

DAY 13

Breakfast
1 frozen waffle
1 c. orange juice
1 T. sugar-free syrup
additional beverage of choice

Lunch
tuna salad sandwich (¼ c. tuna
    salad, 2 sl. bread, 1 sl.
    reduced-fat cheese, sliced
    tomato/romaine lettuce)
1 c. raw vegetables
1 pear
½ c. skim milk
additional beverage of choice

Dinner
3 oz. grilled beef sirloin
½ c. grilled mushrooms
1 medium baked potato
1 T. fat-free sour cream
Stuffed Tomato
¾ c. pineapple
1 small dinner roll

Snack
1 c. fat-free yogurt (artificially
    sweetened)
1½ c. low-fat popcorn

DAY 14

Breakfast
1 c. fat-free yogurt (artificially
    sweetened)
½ c. sliced peaches
1 bagel
1 T. reduced-fat cream cheese
beverage of choice

Lunch
low-fat hot dog on bun
¼ c. baked beans
1 c. raw vegetables
2 T. fat-free ranch dressing
¼ c. low-fat cottage cheese
beverage of choice

Dinner
Stuffed Chicken Popover
1 c. zucchini/carrots
1 c. Caesar salad
2 T. fat-free Caesar salad dressing
Fruit Pizza
beverage of choice

Snack
1 banana with 2 t. peanut butter
½ c. skim milk

DAY 15

Breakfast
2 **Ham and Cheese Muffins**

1 orange
beverage of choice

Lunch
4 oz. roast turkey
2 T. fat-free gravy
Sweet Potato on the Half Shell
1 c. brussels sprouts
½ small dinner roll
beverage of choice

Dinner
2 sl. thin-crust pizza
1 c. vegetable salad
2 T. fat-free salad dressing
1 soft bread stick
1 plum
beverage of choice

Snack
½ serving **Orange Cream
    Smoothie**

DAY 16

Breakfast
¾ c. cold cereal (unsweetened)
1 c. skim milk
½ c. orange or apple juice
additional beverage of choice

Lunch
Greek Couscous Salad
1 c. raw baby carrots
1 pc. string cheese
5 sl. melba toast
beverage of choice

Dinner
Pork Stroganoff
1 c. cooked mixed vegetables
1 c. vegetable salad
2 T. low-fat dressing
1 c. melon balls
1 sl. whole-wheat bread
1 t. butter
beverage of choice

Snack
Berry Banana Smoothie

DAY 17

Breakfast
1 c. fat-free yogurt (artificially
    sweetened)
1 c. raspberries
1 scrambled egg
beverage of choice

Lunch
Cheese Tortellini Soup
1 c. raw vegetables
2 T. low-fat ranch dressing
24 oyster crackers
beverage of choice

Dinner
spaghetti with meat sauce
    (1 c. pasta, 1 c. sauce)
1 c. vegetable salad
2 T. low-fat salad dressing
1 soft bread stick
1 small apple
beverage of choice

Snack
1 c. sugar-free pudding

DAY 18

Breakfast
2 sl. raisin toast (unfrosted)
1 t. butter
½ c. apple juice
additional beverage of choice

Lunch
deli plate (2 oz. lean deli meat, 1½
    oz. reduced-fat cheese, 1 sliced
    orange, 1 c. raw vegetables)
2 small whole-wheat rolls
beverage of choice

Dinner
**Chicken Enchilada in White Cream
    Sauce**
Mexican Cornbread
1½ c. cooked green beans
1 t. butter
½ c. fruit salad
beverage of choice

Snack
15 grapes
3 graham cracker squares

DAY 19

Breakfast
¾ c. cold cereal
½ c. skim milk
½ grapefruit
beverage of choice

Lunch
grilled cheese sandwich
Apple Carrot Salad
1 c. vegetable salad
2 T. fat-free salad dressing
1 small muffin
beverage of choice

Dinner
4 oz. meatloaf
Creamy Mashed Potatoes
2 T. fat-free gravy
1 c. cooked carrots
1 nectarine
1 sl. whole-wheat bread
beverage of choice

Snack
½ c. frozen vanilla yogurt

DAY 20

Breakfast
1 c. oatmeal
1 c. skim milk
½ c. orange juice
additional beverage of choice

Lunch
large vegetable salad
¼ c. fat-free dressing
2 small rolls
1 t. butter
beverage of choice

Dinner
2 **Grilled Fish Tacos**
½ c. cooked zucchini
beverage of choice

Snack
Cherry Almond Smoothie
1 granola bar

DAY 21

Breakfast
1 English muffin
1 c. berries
1 t. butter
beverage of choice

Lunch
Baked Potato Soup
2 c. raw vegetables
2 T. fat-free ranch dressing
¾ c. pineapple
beverage of choice

Dinner
2 **Pizza Burgers**
1 c. cooked mixed vegetables
beverage of choice

Snack
½ c. fat-free yogurt (artificially
    sweetened)
¾ c. peach slices

DAY 22

Breakfast
1 bagel
1 T. cream cheese
1 c. juice blend
additional beverage of choice

Lunch
Hashbrown Quiche
Melon Berry Soup
2 c. vegetable salad
2 T. fat-free salad dressing
1 soft bread stick
beverage of choice

Dinner
3 oz. barbecued beef on bun
½ c. baked beans
1 c. raw baby carrots
2 T. low-fat ranch dressing
beverage of choice

Snack
Piña Colada Smoothie

DAY 23

Breakfast
1½ c. cold cereal
    (unsweetened)
1 c. skim milk
½ c. orange juice

Lunch
Chicken Enchilada Soup
1 c. vegetable salad
2 T. low-fat salad dressing
¼ c. low-fat cottage cheese
½ c. fruit cocktail
    (unsweetened)
6 whole-wheat crackers
beverage of choice

Dinner
Creamy Sausage Creole
½ c. cooked green beans with
    1 T. almonds
beverage of choice

Snack
Berry Berry Berry Smoothie

DAY 24

Breakfast
1 c. fat-free yogurt (artificially
    sweetened)
¾ c. blueberries
¼ c. fat-free granola
beverage of choice

Lunch
  beef and cheese quesadilla
    (1½ oz. reduced-fat cheese,
    2 oz. cooked ground beef, two
    6" flour tortillas)
  1 sliced tomato
  2 T. fat-free sour cream
  salsa
  beverage of choice

Dinner
  2 sl. **Reuben Pizza**
  2 c. vegetable salad
  ½ c. cooked mixed vegetables
  1 peach
  beverage of choice

Snack
  2 watermelon wedges
  1 sl. of bread with 2 T. peanut
    butter

DAY 25

Breakfast
  1 English muffin
  2 t. butter
  beverage of choice

Lunch
  **Grilled Turkey, Vegetable, and
    Cheese Sandwich**
  ½ c. cooked spinach
  ½ c. tomato/vegetable juice
  beverage of choice

Dinner
  3 oz. baked salmon fillet
  ½ c. green peas
  1 c. cooked carrots
  ½ c. skim milk
  ½ c. applesauce (unsweetened)
  2 sl. whole-wheat bread
  additional beverage of choice

Snack
  Tropical Smoothie

DAY 26

Breakfast
  1 c. cooked cereal
  ½ c. skim milk
  ½ c. orange juice
  additional beverage of choice

Lunch
  1 c. chili/beans with 2 oz. reduced-
    fat cheese
  1 c. raw vegetables
  2 T. fat-free ranch dressing
  24 oyster crackers
  beverage of choice

Dinner
  Stromboli
  1 c. cooked broccoli/cauliflower
  1 c. berries
  beverage of choice

Snack
  Creamy Peach Smoothie

DAY 27

Breakfast
  1½ c. cold cereal (unsweetened)
  1 c. skim milk
  1 banana
  beverage of choice

Lunch
  Caesar Tortellini Salad
  ¼ c. low-fat croutons
  1 T. sunflower seeds
  1 orange
  beverage of choice

Dinner
  2 oz. grilled pork chop
  1½ c. grilled vegetables
  1 baked apple
  2 small dinner rolls
  beverage of choice

Snack
  1 c. sugar-free pudding

DAY 28

Breakfast
yogurt/fruit parfait (½ c. artificially
   sweetened fat-free yogurt and
   1 c. berries)
⅓ c. Grape Nuts cereal (sprinkled
   over parfait)
beverage of choice

Lunch
Chef's Pasta Salad
1 c. melon balls
1 c. tomato/vegetable juice

1 c. raw baby carrots
beverage of choice

Dinner
Fajita Lettuce Wrap
2 T. fat-free sour cream
½ c. canned fruit (unsweetened)
½ large ear corn on the cob
beverage of choice

Snack
1 sl. bread with 2 T. peanut butter
1 pear

2000-Calorie Calcium Key Meal Plans

DAY 1

Breakfast
2 sl. **Baked French Toast with
   Maple Yogurt and Fruit**
beverage of choice

Lunch
3 oz. roasted chicken
1 medium baked potato
2 T. fat-free sour cream
1 c. melon balls
1 c. mixed vegetables
1 dinner roll
1 t. butter
beverage of choice

Dinner
2 sl. cheese pizza
1 c. raw vegetables
¾ c. pineapple
beverage of choice

Snack
½ c. sugar-free pudding

DAY 2

Breakfast
¾ c. cold cereal (unsweetened)

½ c. skim milk
½ c. orange juice
1 hard-cooked egg
1 sl. whole-wheat toast
1 t. butter
additional beverage of choice

Lunch
1 pc. string cheese
12 whole-wheat crackers
**Fresh Fruit Kebob with Citrus
   Poppy-Seed Dressing**
1 c. raw broccoli/cauliflower
beverage of choice

Dinner
Turkey Tet-rotini
1½ c. cooked carrots
lettuce salad
2 T. low-fat salad dressing
1 c. strawberries
1 small dinner roll
1 t. butter
beverage of choice

Snack
1 oz. turkey
1 sl. whole-wheat bread
1 orange

DAY 3

Breakfast
2 sl. whole-wheat toast
1 t. butter
½ c. orange juice
additional beverage of choice

Lunch
Tuna Cheese Salad
vegetable salad
2 T. low-fat salad dressing
1 peach
½ c. tomato juice
1 sl. rye bread
1 t. butter
additional beverage of choice

Dinner
Mediterranean Lentil Soup
1 c. raw vegetables
2 T. fat-free ranch dressing
9 whole-wheat crackers
beverage of choice

Snack
Berry Blue Smoothie
3 squares graham crackers

DAY 4

Breakfast
1 c. oatmeal
½ c. skim milk
1 tangerine
beverage of choice

Lunch
cheeseburger (4 oz. meat, 1 sl.
    cheese, 1 bun, lettuce, tomato,
    onion)
1 T. low-fat mayonnaise
Potato Salad
1 c. raw vegetable sticks
1 watermelon wedge
beverage of choice

Dinner
Eggplant Lasagna
vegetable salad
2 T. low-fat salad dressing
½ c. fruit salad
2 sl. French bread
2 t. butter
1/12 angel food cake
beverage of choice

Snack
½ c. flavored fat-free yogurt
1 small apple

DAY 5

Breakfast
1 bagel
1 T. cream cheese
½ c. orange juice
additional beverage of choice

Lunch
Pita Shrimp
1 c. raw vegetables
1 T. low-fat dressing
2 plums
2 squares graham crackers
beverage of choice

Dinner
3 oz. roast/grilled pork
    tenderloin
Creamy Spring Risotto
2 sl. bread
1 t. butter
beverage of choice

Snack
Berry Berry Berry Smoothie
3 c. low-fat popcorn

DAY 6

Breakfast
 2 **Tammi's Minnesota Muffins**
 ½ grapefruit
 beverage of choice

Lunch
 ½ c. low-fat cottage cheese
 2 canned peach halves in juice
 2 oz. deli lean ham/turkey
 1 c. vegetable salad
 2 T. fat-free salad dressing
 2 soft bread sticks
 beverage of choice

Dinner
 **Portabella Mushroom Burger with
 Caramelized Balsamic Onions**
 lettuce and tomato slices
 1 T. low-fat mayonnaise
 6 spears grilled asparagus
 2 c. berries
 3 ginger snaps
 beverage of choice

Snack
 Piña Colada Smoothie
 1 granola bar

DAY 7

Breakfast
 ¾ c. cold cereal (unsweetened)
 1 c. skim milk
 1 small banana
 1 sl. whole-wheat toast
 1 t. butter
 beverage of choice

Lunch
 Wild Rice Soup
 9 whole-wheat crackers
 Frozen Fruit Cup
 beverage of choice

Dinner
 chicken and vegetable stir-fry
 (3 oz. chicken, 1½ c.
 vegetables)

1 c. cooked brown rice
⅛ honeydew melon
beverage of choice

Snack
 1 apple with 2 t. peanut butter
 ¾ c. small pretzel twists

DAY 8

Breakfast
 2 **Sautéed Apple Crepes**
 1 c. skim milk
 additional beverage of choice

Lunch
 4 oz. lean baked ham
 1 c. cooked asparagus
 lettuce salad
 2 T. low-fat salad dressing
 ¾ c. peach slices
 1 small dinner roll
 beverage of choice

Dinner
 Tomato Pepper Penne
 1 c. raw vegetables
 2 T. low-fat ranch dressing
 15 grapes
 2 sl. French bread
 1 t. butter
 beverage of choice

Snack
 1 orange
 6 squares graham crackers

DAY 9

Breakfast
 2 English muffins
 ½ c. fat-free yogurt (artificially
 sweetened)
 ½ banana
 1 t. butter
 beverage of choice

Lunch
 Fruit and Cheese Salad

2 sl. whole-wheat bread
1 c. coleslaw (made with fat-free
    dressing)
beverage of choice

Dinner
4 oz. grilled chicken
Tabbouleh Zucchini
1 c. corn
lettuce salad
2 T. fat-free salad dressing
1 sl. whole-wheat bread
beverage of choice

Snack
Cherry Almond Smoothie
1 c. raw baby carrots

DAY 10

Breakfast
1 c. cold cereal (unsweetened)
½ c. skim milk
1 hard-cooked egg
1 sl. whole-wheat toast
1 t. butter
beverage of choice

Lunch
Oriental Chicken Salad
6 sl. melba toast
1 t. butter
12 animal crackers
½ c. sliced strawberries
beverage of choice

Dinner
Chili Cheese Casserole
1 c. cooked broccoli
1 c. vegetable salad
2 T. fat-free salad dressing
2-inch-square cornbread
1 watermelon wedge
beverage of choice

Snack
Grape Ape Smoothie
1 fat-free granola bar

DAY 11

Breakfast
yogurt/fruit parfait (1 c. artificially
    sweetened nonfat yogurt and
    1 c. berries)
3 T. Grape Nuts cereal (sprinkled
    over parfait)
beverage of choice

Lunch
Veggie and Cheese Sub Sandwich
2 tangerines
beverage of choice

Dinner
2 c. beef stew
2 small biscuits
1 t. butter
1 c. sliced cucumber
½ c. canned fruit (unsweetened)
beverage of choice

Snack
1 c. pudding (artificially sweetened)
3 squares graham crackers

DAY 12

Breakfast
1 c. cooked cereal
1 c. skim milk
½ grapefruit
beverage of choice

Lunch
taco with meat and cheese
⅔ c. Spanish rice
1 sliced tomato
½ c. unsweetened applesauce
beverage of choice

Dinner
Parmesan Roughy
1 c. green beans with 2 T. almonds
1 c. buttered noodles
2 sl. rye bread
1 t. butter
beverage of choice

Snack
Fuzzy Berry Smoothie
3 vanilla wafers

DAY 13

Breakfast
2 frozen waffles
2 T. sugar-free syrup
1 c. orange juice
additional beverage of choice

Lunch
tuna salad sandwich (¼ c. tuna
    salad, 2 sl. bread, 1 sl.
    reduced-fat cheese, sliced
    tomato/romaine lettuce)
1 c. raw vegetables
1 pear
½ c. skim milk
additional beverage of choice

Dinner
3 oz. grilled beef sirloin
½ c. grilled mushrooms
1 medium baked potato
1 T. fat-free sour cream
Stuffed Tomato
¾ c. pineapple
2 small dinner rolls

Snack
1 c. fat-free yogurt (artificially
    sweetened)
1½ c. low-fat popcorn

DAY 14

Breakfast
1 c. fat-free yogurt (artificially
    sweetened)
½ c. sliced peaches
1 bagel
3 T. reduced-fat cream cheese
beverage of choice

Lunch
low-fat hot dog on bun
½ c. baked beans
1 c. raw vegetables
2 T. fat-free ranch dressing
¼ c. low-fat cottage cheese
beverage of choice

Dinner
Stuffed Chicken Popover
1 c. zucchini/carrots
1 c. Caesar salad
2 T. fat-free Caesar salad dressing
Fruit Pizza
beverage of choice

Snack
½ c. skim milk
1 fat-free granola bar
1 banana with 2 t. peanut butter

DAY 15

Breakfast
2 Ham and Cheese Muffins
1 orange
beverage of choice

Lunch
4 oz. roast turkey
2 T. fat-free gravy
Sweet Potato on the Half Shell
1 c. brussels sprouts
1½ small dinner roll
1 t. butter
beverage of choice

Dinner
2 sl. thin-crust pizza
1 c. vegetable salad
2 T. fat-free salad dressing
1 soft bread stick
1 plum
beverage of choice

Snack
½ serving **Orange Cream Smoothie**
3 squares graham crackers

DAY 16

Breakfast
¾ c. cold cereal (unsweetened)
1 sl. whole-wheat toast
1 t. butter
½ c. skim milk
½ c. orange or apple juice
additional beverage of choice

Lunch
Greek Couscous Salad
1 c. raw baby carrots
1 pc. string cheese
5 sl. melba toast
beverage of choice

Dinner
Pork Stroganoff
1 c. cooked mixed vegetables
1 c. vegetable salad
2 T. low-fat dressing
1 c. melon balls
1 sl. whole-wheat bread
1 t. butter
beverage of choice

Snack
Berry Banana Smoothie

DAY 17

Breakfast
1 c. fat-free yogurt (artificially
  sweetened)
1 c. raspberries
1 scrambled egg
1 sl. whole-wheat toast
1 t. butter
beverage of choice

Lunch
Cheese Tortellini Soup
1 c. raw vegetables
2 T. low-fat ranch dressing
24 oyster crackers
beverage of choice

Dinner
spaghetti with meat sauce
  (1½ c. pasta, 1 c. sauce)
1 c. vegetable salad
2 T. low-fat salad dressing
1 soft bread stick
1 small apple
beverage of choice

Snack
1 c. sugar-free pudding

DAY 18

Breakfast
2 sl. raisin toast (unfrosted)
1 t. butter
½ c. apple juice
additional beverage of choice

Lunch
deli plate (2 oz. lean deli meat,
  1½ oz. reduced-fat cheese,
  1 sliced orange, 1 c. raw
  vegetables)
2 small whole-wheat rolls
6 vanilla wafers
beverage of choice

Dinner
**Chicken Enchilada in White Cream
  Sauce**
Mexican Cornbread
1½ c. cooked green beans
1 t. butter
½ c. fruit salad
beverage of choice

Snack
15 grapes
6 graham cracker squares

DAY 19

Breakfast
¾ c. cold cereal (unsweetened)
½ c. skim milk
½ grapefruit
beverage of choice

Lunch
grilled cheese sandwich
Apple Carrot Salad
1 c. vegetable salad
2 T. fat-free salad dressing
2 small muffins
1 t. butter
beverage of choice

Dinner
4 oz. meatloaf
Creamy Mashed Potatoes
2 T. fat-free gravy
1 c. cooked carrots
1 nectarine
2 sl. whole-wheat bread
beverage of choice

Snack
½ c. frozen vanilla yogurt

DAY 20

Breakfast
1 c. oatmeal
1 c. skim milk
½ c. orange juice
additional beverage of choice

Lunch
large vegetable salad
¼ c. fat-free dressing
2 small rolls
2 t. butter
1/12 angel food cake
beverage of choice

Dinner
2 **Grilled Fish Tacos**
½ c. cooked zucchini
beverage of choice

Snack
Cherry Almond Smoothie
1 granola bar

DAY 21

Breakfast
1 English muffin
1 c. berries
1 t. butter
beverage of choice

Lunch
Baked Potato Soup
2 c. raw vegetables
2 T. low-fat ranch dressing
¾ c. pineapple
6 whole-wheat crackers
beverage of choice

Dinner
2 **Pizza Burgers**
1 c. cooked mixed vegetables
½ c. canned fruit
   (unsweetened)
beverage of choice

Snack
½ c. fat-free yogurt (artificially
   sweetened)
¾ c. peach slices

DAY 22

Breakfast
1 bagel
2 T. cream cheese
1 c. juice blend
additional beverage of choice

Lunch
Hashbrown Quiche
Melon Berry Soup
2 c. vegetable salad
2 T. fat-free salad dressing
2 soft bread sticks
beverage of choice

Dinner
3 oz. barbecued beef on bun
½ c. baked beans
1 c. raw baby carrots
2 T. low-fat ranch dressing
beverage of choice

Snack
Piña Colada Smoothie
3 squares graham crackers

DAY 23

Breakfast
1½ c. cold cereal (unsweetened)
1 c. skim milk
½ c. orange juice
additional beverage of choice

Lunch
Chicken Enchilada Soup
1 c. vegetable salad
2 T. low-fat salad dressing
¼ c. low-fat cottage cheese
½ c. fruit cocktail (unsweetened)
6 whole-wheat crackers
beverage of choice

Dinner
Creamy Sausage Creole
½ c. cooked green beans with 2 T.
almonds
1 sl. whole-wheat bread
1 t. butter
beverage of choice

Snack
Berry Berry Berry Smoothie
1 fat-free granola bar

DAY 24

Breakfast
1 c. fat-free yogurt (artificially
sweetened)
¾ c. blueberries
½ c. fat-free granola
beverage of choice

Lunch
beef and cheese quesadilla
(1½ oz. reduced-fat cheese,
2 oz. cooked ground beef, two
6" flour tortillas)
1 sliced tomato
2 T. fat-free sour cream
salsa
beverage of choice

Dinner
2 sl. **Reuben Pizza**
2 c. vegetable salad
½ c. cooked mixed vegetables
1 peach
beverage of choice

Snack
2 watermelon wedges
2 sl. of bread with 2½ T. peanut
butter

DAY 25

Breakfast
2 English muffins
2 t. butter
beverage of choice

Lunch
**Grilled Turkey, Vegetable, and
Cheese Sandwich**
½ c. cooked spinach
½ c. tomato/vegetable juice
additional beverage of choice

Dinner
3 oz. baked salmon fillet
½ c. cooked peas
1 c. cooked carrots
½ c. skim milk
½ c. applesauce (unsweetened)
2 sl. whole-wheat bread
1 t. butter
additional beverage of choice

Snack
Tropical Smoothie

DAY 26

Breakfast
1 c. cooked cereal
½ c. skim milk
½ c. orange juice
additional beverage of choice

Lunch
1 c. chili/beans with 2 oz.
reduced-fat cheese
1 c. raw vegetables
2 T. fat-free ranch dressing
24 oyster crackers
beverage of choice

Dinner
Stromboli
1 c. cooked broccoli/cauliflower
1 c. berries
1 sl. garlic toast
beverage of choice

Snack
Creamy Peach Smoothie
3 c. low-fat popcorn

DAY 27

Breakfast
1½ c. cold cereal
(unsweetened)
1 c. skim milk
1 banana
beverage of choice

Lunch
Caesar Tortellini Salad
¼ c. low-fat croutons
1 T. sunflower seeds
1 orange
5 sl. melba toast
beverage of choice

Dinner
2 oz. grilled pork chop
1½ c. grilled vegetables
1 baked apple
2 small dinner rolls
1 t. butter
beverage of choice

Snack
1 c. sugar-free pudding
3 ginger snaps

DAY 28

Breakfast
yogurt/fruit parfait (½ c. artificially
sweetened nonfat yogurt and
1 c. berries)
⅓ c. Grape Nuts cereal (sprinkled
over parfait)
beverage of choice

Lunch
Chef's Pasta Salad
1 c. melon balls
1 c. tomato/vegetable juice
6 fat-free whole-wheat crackers
1 c. raw baby carrots
additional beverage of choice

Dinner
Fajita Lettuce Wrap
2 T. fat-free sour cream
½ c. canned fruit (unsweetened)
1 large ear corn on the cob
1 t. butter
beverage of choice

Snack
1 sl. bread with 2 T. peanut
butter
1 pear

2200-Calorie Calcium Key Meal Plans

DAY 1

Breakfast
2 sl. **Baked French Toast with Maple Yogurt and Fruit**
beverage of choice

Lunch
3 oz. roasted chicken
1 medium baked potato
2 T. fat-free sour cream
1 c. melon balls
1½ c. mixed vegetables
1 dinner roll
1 t. butter
beverage of choice

Dinner
2 sl. cheese pizza
1 c. raw vegetables
¾ c. pineapple
beverage of choice

Snack
½ c. sugar-free pudding
granola bar

DAY 2

Breakfast
¾ c. cold cereal (unsweetened)
½ c. skim milk
½ c. orange juice
1 hard-cooked egg
1 sl. whole-wheat toast
1 t. butter
additional beverage of choice

Lunch
1 pc. string cheese
12 whole-wheat crackers
Fresh Fruit Kebob with Citrus Poppy-Seed Dressing
1 c. raw broccoli/cauliflower
1 cucumber, sliced
beverage of choice

Dinner
Turkey Tet-rotini
1½ c. cooked carrots
lettuce salad
2 T. low-fat salad dressing
1 c. strawberries
1 small dinner roll
1 t. butter
beverage of choice

Snack
1 oz. turkey
1 t. low-fat mayonnaise
2 sl. whole-wheat bread
1 orange

DAY 3

Breakfast
2 sl. whole-wheat toast
2 t. butter
½ c. orange juice
additional beverage of choice

Lunch
Tuna Cheese Salad
vegetable salad
2 T. low-fat salad dressing
1 peach
½ c. tomato juice
1 sl. rye bread
1 t. butter
additional beverage of choice

Dinner
Mediterranean Lentil Soup
2 c. raw vegetables
2 T. fat-free ranch dressing
9 whole-wheat crackers
beverage of choice

Snack
Berry Blue Smoothie
6 squares graham crackers

DAY 4

Breakfast
- 1 c. oatmeal
- ½ c. skim milk
- 1 tangerine
- beverage of choice

Lunch
- cheeseburger (4 oz. meat, 1 sl. cheese, 1 bun, lettuce, tomato, onion)
- 1 T. low-fat mayonnaise
- **Potato Salad**
- 1 c. raw vegetable sticks
- 1 watermelon wedge
- beverage of choice

Dinner
- **Eggplant Lasagna**
- vegetable salad
- 2 T. low-fat salad dressing
- ½ c. fruit salad
- 2 sl. French bread
- 2 t. butter
- ¹⁄₁₂ angel food cake
- beverage of choice

Snack
- ½ c. flavored fat-free yogurt
- 1 small apple
- 3 squares graham crackers

DAY 5

Breakfast
- 1 bagel
- 1½ T. cream cheese
- ½ c. orange juice
- additional beverage of choice

Lunch
- **Pita Shrimp**
- 1 c. raw vegetables
- 2 T. low-fat dressing
- 2 plums
- 5 squares graham crackers
- beverage of choice

Dinner
- 3 oz. roast/grilled pork tenderloin
- **Creamy Spring Risotto**
- 2 sl. bread
- 1 t. butter
- beverage of choice

Snack
- **Berry Berry Berry Smoothie**
- 3 c. low-fat popcorn

DAY 6

Breakfast
- 2 **Tammi's Minnesota Muffins**
- ½ grapefruit
- beverage of choice

Lunch
- ½ c. low-fat cottage cheese
- 2 canned peach halves in juice
- 2 oz. deli lean ham/turkey
- 1½ c. vegetable salad
- 2 T. low-fat salad dressing
- 2 soft bread sticks
- beverage of choice

Dinner
- **Portabella Mushroom Burger with Caramelized Balsamic Onions**
- lettuce and tomato slices
- 1 T. low-fat mayonnaise
- 9 spears grilled asparagus
- 2 c. berries
- 6 ginger snaps
- beverage of choice

Snack
- **Piña Colada Smoothie**
- 1 granola bar

DAY 7

Breakfast
- ¾ c. cold cereal (unsweetened)
- 1 c. skim milk
- 1 small banana
- 2 sl. whole-wheat toast
- 2 t. butter
- beverage of choice

Lunch
Wild Rice Soup
9 whole-wheat crackers
Frozen Fruit Cup
1 c. carrot/celery sticks
beverage of choice

Dinner
chicken and vegetable stir-fry
(3 oz. chicken, 1½ c.
vegetables)
1 c. cooked brown rice
⅛ honeydew melon
beverage of choice

Snack
1 apple with 2 t. peanut butter
¾ c. small pretzel twists

DAY 8

Breakfast
2 **Sautéed Apple Crepes**
1 c. skim milk
½ c. tomato/vegetable juice
additional beverage of choice

Lunch
4 oz. lean baked ham
1 c. cooked asparagus
lettuce salad
2 T. low-fat salad dressing
¾ c. peach slices
2 small dinner rolls
1 t. butter
beverage of choice

Dinner
Tomato Pepper Penne
1 c. raw vegetables
2 T. low-fat ranch dressing
15 grapes
2 sl. French bread
1 t. butter
beverage of choice

Snack
1 orange
6 squares graham crackers

DAY 9

Breakfast
2 English muffins
½ c. nonfat yogurt (artificially
sweetened)
½ banana
1 t. butter
beverage of choice

Lunch
Fruit and Cheese Salad
2 sl. whole-wheat bread
1 c. coleslaw (made with fat-free
dressing)
1 t. butter
¹⁄₁₂ angel food cake
beverage of choice

Dinner
4 oz. grilled chicken
Tabbouleh Zucchini
1 c. corn
lettuce salad
2 T. fat-free salad dressing
2 sl. whole-wheat bread
beverage of choice

Snack
Cherry Almond Smoothie
1 c. raw baby carrots

DAY 10

Breakfast
1 c. cold cereal (unsweetened)
½ c. skim milk
1 hard-cooked egg
1 sl. whole-wheat toast
1 t. butter
beverage of choice

Lunch
Oriental Chicken Salad
6 sl. melba toast
1 t. butter
12 animal crackers
½ c. sliced strawberries
½ c. tomato/vegetable juice
additional beverage of choice

Dinner
Chili Cheese Casserole
1 c. cooked broccoli
1 c. vegetable salad
2 T. fat-free salad dressing
2-inch-square cornbread
1 watermelon wedge
beverage of choice

Snack
Grape Ape Smoothie
fat-free granola bar

DAY 11

Breakfast
yogurt/fruit parfait (1 c. nonfat
    artificially sweetened yogurt and
    1 c. berries)
3 T. Grape Nuts cereal (sprinkled
    over parfait)
beverage of choice

Lunch
Veggie and Cheese Sub Sandwich
2 tangerines
1 c. vegetable salad
2 T. low-fat salad dressing
½ c. croutons
beverage of choice

Dinner
2 c. beef stew
2 small biscuits
1 t. butter
1 c. sliced cucumber
½ c. canned fruit (unsweetened)
beverage of choice

Snack
1 c. pudding (artificially sweetened)
3 squares graham crackers

DAY 12

Breakfast
1¼ c. cooked cereal
1 c. skim milk
½ grapefruit
beverage of choice

Lunch
taco with meat and cheese
⅔ c. Spanish rice
1 sliced tomato
½ c. unsweetened applesauce
beverage of choice

Dinner
Parmesan Roughy
1 c. green beans with 2 T. almonds
1 c. buttered noodles
½ c. coleslaw (made with fat-free
    dressing)
2 sl. rye bread
1 t. butter
beverage of choice

Snack
Fuzzy Berry Smoothie
6 vanilla wafers

DAY 13

Breakfast
2 frozen waffles
1 c. orange juice
2 T. sugar-free syrup
additional beverage of choice

Lunch
tuna salad sandwich (¼ c. tuna
    salad, 2 sl. bread, 1 sl.
    reduced-fat cheese, sliced
    tomato/romaine lettuce)
1 c. raw vegetables
1 pear
½ c. skim milk
½ c. tomato/vegetable juice
additional beverage of choice

Dinner
3 oz. grilled beef sirloin
½ c. grilled mushrooms
1 large baked potato
1 T. fat-free sour cream
Stuffed Tomato
¾ c. pineapple
2 small dinner rolls
1 t. butter
beverage of choice

Snack
- 1 c. fat-free yogurt (artificially sweetened)
- 3 c. low-fat popcorn

DAY 14

Breakfast
- 1 c. fat-free yogurt (artificially sweetened)
- ½ c. sliced peaches
- 1 bagel
- 3 T. reduced-fat cream cheese
- beverage of choice

Lunch
- low-fat hot dog on bun
- ½ c. baked beans
- 1 c. raw vegetables
- 2 T. fat-free ranch dressing
- ¼ c. low-fat cottage cheese
- 3 ginger snaps
- beverage of choice

Dinner
- **Stuffed Chicken Popover**
- 1 c. zucchini/carrots
- 1 c. Caesar salad
- 2 T. fat-free Caesar salad dressing
- **Fruit Pizza**
- beverage of choice

Snack
- 1 banana with 2 t. peanut butter
- 1 granola bar
- ½ c. skim milk

DAY 15

Breakfast
- 2 **Ham and Cheese Muffins**
- 1 orange
- ½ c. tomato/vegetable juice
- beverage of choice

Lunch
- 4 oz. roast turkey
- 2 T. fat-free gravy

Sweet Potato on the Half Shell
- 1 c. brussels sprouts
- 1½ small dinner roll
- 1 t. butter
- beverage of choice

Dinner
- 2 sl. thin-crust pizza
- 1 c. vegetable salad
- 2 T. fat-free salad dressing
- 2 soft bread sticks
- 1 t. butter
- 1 plum
- beverage of choice

Snack
- ½ serving **Orange Cream Smoothie**
- 3 squares graham crackers

DAY 16

Breakfast
- ¾ c. cold cereal (unsweetened)
- 1 sl. whole-wheat toast
- 1 t. butter
- ½ c. skim milk
- ½ c. orange or apple juice
- additional beverage of choice

Lunch
- **Greek Couscous Salad**
- 1 c. raw baby carrots
- 1 sliced tomato
- 1 pc. string cheese
- 5 sl. melba toast
- beverage of choice

Dinner
- **Pork Stroganoff**
- 1 c. cooked mixed vegetables
- 1 c. vegetable salad
- 2 T. low-fat dressing
- 1 c. melon balls
- 1 sl. whole-wheat bread
- 1 t. butter
- beverage of choice

Snack
- **Berry Banana Smoothie**
- 1 granola bar

DAY 17

Breakfast
1 c. fat-free yogurt (artificially
    sweetened)
1 c. raspberries
1 scrambled egg
2 sl. whole-wheat toast
2 t. butter
beverage of choice

Lunch
Cheese Tortellini Soup
1 c. raw vegetables
2 T. low-fat ranch dressing
24 oyster crackers
beverage of choice

Dinner
spaghetti with meat sauce
    (1½ c. pasta, 1 c. sauce)
2 c. vegetable salad
2 T. low-fat salad dressing
1 soft bread stick
1 small apple
beverage of choice

Snack
1 c. sugar-free pudding

DAY 18

Breakfast
3 sl. raisin toast (unfrosted)
2 t. butter
½ c. apple juice
additional beverage of choice

Lunch
deli plate (2 oz. lean deli meat, 1½
    oz. reduced-fat cheese, 1 sliced
    orange, 2 c. raw vegetables)
2 small whole-wheat rolls
6 vanilla wafers
beverage of choice

Dinner
**Chicken Enchilada in White Cream
    Sauce**
Mexican Cornbread
1½ c. cooked green beans

1 t. butter
½ c. fruit salad
beverage of choice

Snack
15 grapes
6 graham cracker squares

DAY 19

Breakfast
¾ c. unsweetened cold cereal
½ c. skim milk
½ grapefruit
1 sl. toast
1 t. butter
beverage of choice

Lunch
grilled cheese sandwich
Apple Carrot Salad
1 c. vegetable salad
2 T. fat-free salad dressing
2 small muffins
1 t. butter
beverage of choice

Dinner
4 oz. meatloaf
Creamy Mashed Potatoes
2 T. fat-free gravy
1½ c. cooked carrots
1 nectarine
2 sl. whole-wheat bread
beverage of choice

Snack
½ c. frozen vanilla yogurt

DAY 20

Breakfast
1 c. oatmeal
1 c. skim milk
½ c. orange juice
additional beverage of choice

Lunch
large vegetable salad
¼ c. fat-free dressing

2 small rolls
2 t. butter
1/12 angel food cake
beverage of choice

Dinner
2 Grilled Fish Tacos
1 c. cooked zucchini
10 baked tortilla chips
beverage of choice

Snack
Cherry Almond Smoothie
1 granola bar

DAY 21

Breakfast
1 English muffin
1 c. berries
2 t. butter
beverage of choice

Lunch
Baked Potato Soup
2 c. raw vegetables
2 T. low-fat ranch dressing
3/4 c. pineapple
12 whole-wheat crackers
beverage of choice

Dinner
2 Pizza Burgers
1 c. cooked mixed vegetables
1/2 c. canned fruit (unsweetened)
1/2 c. tomato/vegetable juice
beverage of choice

Snack
1/2 c. fat-free yogurt (artificially
    sweetened)
3/4 c. peach slices

DAY 22

Breakfast
1 bagel
2 T. cream cheese
1 c. juice blend
additional beverage of choice

Lunch
Hashbrown Quiche
Melon Berry Soup
2 c. vegetable salad
2 T. fat-free salad dressing
2 soft bread sticks
1 t. butter
1/2 c. tomato/vegetable juice
beverage of choice

Dinner
3 oz. barbecued beef on bun
3/4 c. baked beans
1 c. raw baby carrots
2 T. low-fat ranch dressing
beverage of choice

Snack
Piña Colada Smoothie
3 squares graham crackers

DAY 23

Breakfast
1 1/2 c. cold cereal (unsweetened)
1 c. skim milk
1/2 c. orange juice
additional beverage of choice

Lunch
Chicken Enchilada Soup
1 c. vegetable salad
2 T. low-fat salad dressing
1/4 c. low-fat cottage cheese
1/2 c. fruit cocktail (unsweetened)
6 whole-wheat crackers
beverage of choice

Dinner
Creamy Sausage Creole
1/2 c. cooked green beans with 1 T.
    almonds
2 sl. whole-wheat bread
2 t. butter
beverage of choice

Snack
Berry Berry Berry Smoothie
1 fat-free granola bar

DAY 24

Breakfast
1 c. fat-free yogurt (artificially
   sweetened)
¾ c. blueberries
½ c. fat-free granola
beverage of choice

Lunch
beef and cheese quesadilla (1½ oz.
   reduced-fat cheese, 2 oz. cooked
   ground beef, two 6" flour tortillas)
1 sliced tomato
2 T. sour cream
salsa
10 baked tortilla chips
beverage of choice

Dinner
2 sl. **Reuben Pizza**
2 c. vegetable salad
½ c. cooked mixed vegetables
1 peach
beverage of choice

Snack
2 sl. of bread with 2½ T. peanut
   butter
2 watermelon wedges

DAY 25

Breakfast
2 English muffins
1 T. butter
beverage of choice

Lunch
**Grilled Turkey, Vegetable, and
   Cheese Sandwich**
½ c. cooked spinach
½ c. tomato/vegetable juice
additional beverage of choice

Dinner
3 oz. baked salmon fillet
½ c. cooked peas
1 c. cooked carrots

½ c. skim milk
½ c. applesauce (unsweetened)
2 sl. whole-wheat bread
1 t. butter
additional beverage of choice

Snack
Tropical Smoothie
8 animal crackers

DAY 26

Breakfast
1 c. cooked cereal
½ c. skim milk
½ c. orange juice
additional beverage of choice

Lunch
1 c. chili/beans with 2 oz.
   reduced-fat cheese
2 c. raw vegetables
2 T. fat-free ranch dressing
24 oyster crackers
beverage of choice

Dinner
Stromboli
1 c. cooked broccoli/cauliflower
1 c. berries
2 sl. garlic toast
beverage of choice

Snack
Creamy Peach Smoothie
3 c. low-fat popcorn

DAY 27

Breakfast
1½ c. cold cereal (unsweetened)
1 c. skim milk
1 banana
beverage of choice

Lunch
Caesar Tortellini Salad
½ c. low-fat croutons

1 T. sunflower seeds
1 orange
8 sl. melba toast
beverage of choice

Dinner
2 oz. grilled pork chop
2 c. grilled vegetables
1 baked apple
2 small dinner rolls
2 t. butter
beverage of choice

Snack
1 c. sugar-free pudding
3 ginger snaps

DAY 28

Breakfast
yogurt/fruit parfait (½ c. artificially
sweetened fat-free yogurt and
1 c. berries)

⅓ c. Grape Nuts cereal (sprinkled
over parfait)
beverage of choice

Lunch
Chef's Pasta Salad
1 c. melon balls
1 c. tomato/vegetable juice
6 fat-free whole-wheat crackers
1 c. raw baby carrots
additional beverage of choice

Dinner
Fajita Lettuce Wrap
2 T. fat-free sour cream
½ c. canned fruit (unsweetened)
½ large ear corn on the cob
2 t. butter
1 sliced cucumber
beverage of choice

Snack
2 sl. bread with 2 T. peanut butter
1 pear

Holiday Meal Plans

HOLIDAY MEAL #1

1200 Calories:
2 oz. roast turkey
½ serving **Creamy Mashed
Potatoes**
2 T. gravy
1 c. green beans with 1 T. almonds
1 dinner roll
1 sl. fruit pie
beverage of choice

Exchanges:
½ dairy, 2 bread/grain,
2 vegetable, 2 fruit,
2 meat/protein, 2 fat

1400 Calories:
3 oz. roast turkey
Creamy Mashed Potatoes
2 T. gravy
1 c. green beans with 1 T. almonds
1 dinner roll
1 sl. fruit pie
beverage of choice

Exchanges:
1 dairy, 3 bread/grain,
2 vegetable, 2 fruit,
3 meat/protein, 2 fat

1600 Calories:
3 oz. roast turkey
Creamy Mashed Potatoes
2 T. gravy
1 c. green beans with 1 T. almonds
1 dinner roll
1 sl. fruit pie
beverage of choice

Exchanges:
1 dairy, 3 bread/grain,
    2 vegetable, 2 fruit,
    3 meat/protein, 2 fat

1800 Calories:
3 oz. roast turkey
Creamy Mashed Potatoes
2 T. gravy
1 c. green beans with 1 T.
    almonds
1 dinner roll
½ c. fruit salad
1 sl. fruit pie
beverage of choice

Exchanges:
1 dairy, 4 bread/grain,
    2 vegetable, 2 fruit,
    3 meat/protein, 2 fat

2000 Calories:
3 oz. roast turkey
Creamy Mashed Potatoes
2 T. gravy
1 c. green beans with 1 T.
    almonds
2 dinner rolls
½ c. fruit salad
1 sl. fruit pie
beverage of choice

Exchanges:
1 dairy, 5 bread/grain,
    2 vegetable, 2 fruit,
    3 meat/protein, 2 fat

2200 Calories:
3 oz. roast turkey
Creamy Mashed Potatoes
2 T. gravy
1 c. green beans with 1 T. almonds
2 dinner rolls
1 t. butter
½ c. fruit salad
1 sl. fruit pie
beverage of choice

Exchanges:
1 dairy, 5 bread/grain,
    2 vegetable, 2 fruit,
    3 meat/protein, 3 fat

HOLIDAY MEAL #2

1200 Calories:
2 oz. roast beef
½ serving **Creamy Spring Risotto**
lettuce salad
2 T. fat-free salad dressing
1 sl. whole-wheat bread
1 t. butter
3-inch-square frosted cake
beverage of choice

Exchanges:
½ dairy, 2 bread/grain,
    2 vegetable, 3 fruit,
    2 meat/protein, 2 fat

1400 Calories:
3 oz. roast beef
Creamy Spring Risotto
lettuce salad
2 T. fat-free salad dressing
1 sl. whole-wheat bread
1 t. butter
3-inch-square frosted cake
beverage of choice

Exchanges:
1 dairy, 3 bread/grain,
    3 vegetable, 3 fruit,
    3 meat/protein, 2 fat

1600 Calories:
  3 oz. roast beef
  Creamy Spring Risotto
  lettuce salad
  2 T. fat-free salad dressing
  1 sl. fresh whole-wheat bread
  1 t. butter
  3-inch-square frosted cake
  beverage of choice

Exchanges:
  1 dairy, 3 bread/grain,
    3 vegetable, 3 fruit,
    3 meat/protein, 2 fat

1800 Calories:
  3 oz. roast beef
  Creamy Spring Risotto
  lettuce salad
  2 T. fat-free salad dressing
  1 sl. fresh whole-wheat bread
  1 t. butter
  **Fresh Fruit Kebob with Citrus
    Poppy-Seed Dressing**
  3-inch-square frosted cake
  beverage of choice

Exchanges:
  1½ dairy, 4½ bread/grain,
    3 vegetable, 3 fruit,
    3 meat/protein, 2 fat

2000 Calories:
  3 oz. roast beef
  Creamy Spring Risotto
  lettuce salad
  2 T. fat-free salad dressing
  2 sl. whole-wheat bread
  1 t. butter
  **Fresh Fruit Kebob with Citrus
    Poppy-Seed Dressing**
  3-inch-square frosted cake
  beverage of choice

Exchanges:
  1½ dairy, 5½ bread/grain,
    3 vegetable, 3 fruit,
    3 meat/protein, 2 fat

2200 Calories:
  3 oz. roast beef
  Creamy Spring Risotto
  lettuce salad
  2 T. fat-free salad dressing
  2 sl. whole-wheat bread
  2 t. butter
  **Fresh Fruit Kebob with Citrus
    Poppy-Seed Dressing**
  3-inch-square frosted cake
  beverage of choice

Exchanges:
  1½ dairy, 5½ bread/grain,
    3 vegetable, 3 fruit,
    3 meat/protein, 3 fat

Restaurant Meal Plans

FAST-FOOD BURGER MEAL

1200 Calories:
  regular cheeseburger on ½ bun
  vegetable salad
  2 T. fat-free salad dressing
  fruit/yogurt parfait
  beverage of choice

Exchanges:
  1½ dairy, 1 bread/grain, 1
    vegetable, 2½ fruit,
    2 meat/protein, 1 fat

1400 Calories:
  regular cheeseburger on bun
  vegetable salad
  2 T. fat-free salad dressing
  fruit/yogurt parfait
  beverage of choice

Exchanges:
  1½ dairy, 2 bread/grain, 1
    vegetable, 2½ fruit,
    2 meat/protein, 1 fat

1600 Calories:
regular cheeseburger on bun
vegetable salad
2 T. fat-free salad dressing
fruit/yogurt parfait
beverage of choice

Exchanges:
1½ dairy, 2 bread/grain,
  1 vegetable, 2½ fruit,
  2 meat/protein, 1 fat

1800 Calories:
regular cheeseburger on bun
1 small french fries
vegetable salad
2 T. fat-free salad dressing
fruit/yogurt parfait
beverage of choice

Exchanges:
1½ dairy, 3½ bread/grain,
  1 vegetable, 2½ fruit,
  2 meat/protein, 2 fat

2000 Calories:
regular cheeseburger on bun
1 small french fries
vegetable salad
2 T. fat-free salad dressing
fruit/yogurt parfait
beverage of choice

Exchanges:
1½ dairy, 3½ bread/grain,
  1 vegetable, 2½ fruit,
  2 meat/protein, 2 fat

2200 Calories:
regular cheeseburger on bun
1 small french fries
vegetable salad
2 T. fat-free salad dressing
fruit/yogurt parfait
beverage of choice

Exchanges:
1½ dairy, 3½ bread/grain,
  1 vegetable, 2½ fruit,
  2 meat/protein, 2 fat

FAST-FOOD CHICKEN MEAL

1200 Calories:
fried chicken leg
½ ear corn on the cob
1 serving macaroni and cheese
vegetable salad
2 T. fat-free salad dressing
beverage of choice

Exchanges:
½ dairy, 2½ bread/grain,
  1 vegetable, 0 fruit,
  2 meat/protein, 1 fat

1400 Calories:
fried chicken thigh or small breast
1 ear corn on the cob
1 serving macaroni and cheese
vegetable salad
2 T. fat-free salad dressing
beverage of choice

Exchanges:
½ dairy, 3½ bread/grain,
  1 vegetable, 0 fruit,
  3 meat/protein, 1 fat

1600 Calories:
fried chicken thigh or small breast
1 ear corn on the cob
1 serving macaroni and cheese
vegetable salad
2 T. fat-free salad dressing
beverage of choice

Exchanges:
½ dairy, 3½ bread/grain,
  1 vegetable, 0 fruit,
  3 meat/protein, 1 fat

1800 Calories:
fried chicken thigh or small
   breast
1 ear corn on the cob
1 serving macaroni and cheese
baked beans
vegetable salad
2 T. fat-free salad dressing
beverage of choice

Exchanges:
½ dairy, 4½ bread/grain,
   1 vegetable, 1 fruit,
   3 meat/protein, 1 fat

2000 Calories:
fried chicken thigh or small
   breast
1 ear corn on the cob
1 serving macaroni and cheese
baked beans
vegetable salad
2 T. fat-free salad dressing
beverage of choice

Exchanges:
½ dairy, 4½ bread/grain,
   1 vegetable, 1 fruit,
   3 meat/protein, 1 fat

2200 Calories:
fried chicken thigh or small
   breast
1 ear corn on the cob
butter
1 serving macaroni and cheese
baked beans
vegetable salad
2 T. fat-free salad dressing
beverage of choice

Exchanges:
½ dairy, 4½ bread/grain,
   1 vegetable, 1 fruit,
   3 meat/protein, 2 fat

SANDWICH/DELI MEAL

1200 Calories:
½ lean meat/cheese 6" sub
1 banana or large apple
beverage of choice

Exchanges:
½ dairy, 1½ bread/grain,
   1 vegetable, 2 fruit,
   1 meat/protein, 1 fat

1400 Calories:
lean meat/cheese 6" sub
1 banana or large apple
beverage of choice

Exchanges:
1 dairy, 3 bread/grain,
   1 vegetable, 2 fruit,
   2 meat/protein, 1 fat

1600 Calories:
lean meat/cheese 6" sub
1 banana or large apple
beverage of choice

Exchanges:
1 dairy, 3 bread/grain,
   1 vegetable, 2 fruit,
   2 meat/protein, 1 fat

1800 Calories:
lean meat/cheese 6" sub
1 banana or large apple
1 oz. baked potato chips
beverage of choice

Exchanges:
1 dairy, 4½ bread/grain,
   1 vegetable, 2 fruit,
   2 meat/protein, 1 fat

2000 Calories:
  lean meat/cheese 6" sub
  1 banana or large apple
  1 oz. baked potato chips
  1 c. cream soup
  beverage of choice

  Exchanges:
  1½ dairy, 5½ bread/grain,
    1 vegetable, 2 fruit,
    2 meat/protein, 2 fat

2200 Calories:
  lean meat/cheese 6" sub
  1 banana or large apple
  1 oz. baked potato chips
  1 c. cream soup
  beverage of choice

  Exchanges:
  1½ dairy, 5½ bread/grain,
    1 vegetable, 2 fruit,
    2 meat/protein, 2 fat

MEXICAN MEAL

1200 Calories:
  chicken soft taco or fajita with
    cheese/salsa
  beverage of choice

  Exchanges:
  1 dairy, 1½ bread/grain,
    1 vegetable, 0 fruit,
    2 meat/protein, 0 fat

1400 Calories:
  chicken soft taco or fajita with
    cheese/salsa
  ⅓ c. Spanish rice
  beverage of choice

  Exchanges:
  1 dairy, 2½ bread/grain,
    1 vegetable, 0 fruit,
    2 meat/protein, 1 fat

1600 Calories:
  chicken soft taco or fajita with
    cheese/salsa
  ⅓ c. Spanish rice
  beverage of choice

  Exchanges:
  1 dairy, 2½ bread/grain,
    1 vegetable, 0 fruit,
    2 meat/protein, 1 fat

1800 Calories:
  chicken soft taco or fajita with
    cheese/salsa
  ⅓ c. Spanish rice
  ½ c. refried beans
  beverage of choice

  Exchanges:
  1 dairy, 4 bread/grain, 1 vegetable,
    0 fruit, 2 meat/protein, 1 fat

2000 Calories:
  chicken soft taco or fajita with
    cheese/salsa
  ⅓ c. Spanish rice
  ½ c. refried beans
  beverage of choice

  Exchanges:
  1 dairy, 4 bread/grain, 1 vegetable,
    0 fruit, 2 meat/protein, 1 fat

2200 Calories:
  chicken soft taco or fajita with
    cheese/salsa
  ⅓ c. Spanish rice
  ½ c. refried beans
  1 oz. tortilla chips
  beverage of choice

  Exchanges:
  1 dairy, 5 bread/grain, 1 vegetable,
    0 fruit, 2 meat/protein, 3 fat

CHINESE MEAL

1200 Calories:
1 c. egg drop soup
stir-fried meat and vegetables (2 oz.
    meat and 1 c. vegetables)
1/3 c. steamed rice
1 fortune cookie
1 orange
beverage of choice

Exchanges:
0 dairy, 2 bread/grain, 2 vegetable,
    1 fruit, 2 meat/protein, 1 fat

1400 Calories:
1 c. egg drop soup
stir-fried meat and vegetables
    (3 oz. meat and 1 c. vegetables)
1/3 c. steamed rice
1 fortune cookie
1 orange
beverage of choice

Exchanges:
0 dairy, 2 bread/grain, 2 vegetable,
    1 fruit, 3 meat/protein, 1 fat

1600 Calories:
1 c. egg drop soup
stir-fried meat and vegetables
    (3 oz. meat and 1 c. vegetables)
1/3 c. steamed rice
1 fortune cookie
1 orange
beverage of choice

Exchanges:
0 dairy, 2 bread/grain, 2 vegetable,
    1 fruit, 3 meat/protein, 1 fat

1800 Calories:
1 c. egg drop soup
stir-fried meat and vegetables
    (3 oz. meat and 1 c. vegetables)
2/3 c. steamed rice
1 fortune cookie
1 orange
beverage of choice

Exchanges:
0 dairy, 3 bread/grain, 2 vegetable,
    1 fruit, 3 meat/protein, 1 fat

2000 Calories:
1 c. egg drop soup
stir-fried meat and vegetables
    (3 oz. meat and 1 c. vegetables)
2/3 c. steamed rice
1 fortune cookie
1 orange
beverage of choice

Exchanges:
0 dairy, 3 bread/grain, 2 vegetable,
    1 fruit, 3 meat/protein, 1 fat

2200 Calories:
1 c. egg drop soup
stir-fried meat and vegetables
    (3 oz. meat and 1 1/2 c.
    vegetables)
1 c. steamed rice
1 fortune cookie
1 orange
beverage of choice

Exchanges:
0 dairy, 4 bread/grain, 3 vegetable,
    1 fruit, 3 meat/protein, 2 fat

BREAKFAST

1200 Calories:
1/2 lite ham/cheese omelet
1 sl. toast
1 c. orange juice
additional beverage of choice

Exchanges:
1/2 dairy, 1 bread/grain,
    0 vegetable, 2 fruit,
    2 meat/protein, 1 fat

1400 Calories:
½ lite ham/cheese omelet
2 sl. toast
1 c. orange juice
additional beverage of choice

Exchanges:
½ dairy, 2 bread/grain,
   0 vegetable, 2 fruit,
   2 meat/protein, 1 fat

1600 Calories:
lite ham/cheese omelet
2 sl. toast
1 c. orange juice
additional beverage of choice

Exchanges:
1 dairy, 2 bread/grain, 0 vegetable,
   2 fruit, 4 meat/protein, 2 fat

1800 Calories:
lite ham/cheese omelet
2 sl. toast
1 t. butter
1 c. orange juice
additional beverage of choice

Exchanges:
1 dairy, 2 bread/grain, 0 vegetable,
   2 fruit, 4 meat/protein, 3 fat

2000 Calories:
lite ham/cheese omelet
2 sl. toast
hash browns
1 c. orange juice
additional beverage of choice

Exchanges:
1 dairy, 3½ bread/grain,
   0 vegetable, 2 fruit,
   4 meat/protein, 3 fat

2200 Calories:
lite ham/cheese omelet
2 sl. toast
hash browns
1½ c. orange juice
additional beverage of choice

Exchanges:
1 dairy, 3½ bread/grain,
   0 vegetable, 3 fruit,
   4 meat/protein, 3 fat

SEAFOOD MEAL

1200 Calories:
1 c. clam chowder
2 oz. baked fish of choice
½ baked potato
2 T. sour cream
vegetable salad
2 T. fat-free salad dressing
beverage of choice

Exchanges:
½ dairy, 2 bread/grain,
   1 vegetable, 0 fruit,
   2 meat/protein, 2 fat

1400 Calories:
1 c. clam chowder
3 oz. baked fish of choice
½ baked potato
2 T. sour cream
vegetable salad
2 T. fat-free salad dressing
beverage of choice

Exchanges:
½ dairy, 2 bread/grain,
   1 vegetable, 0 fruit,
   3 meat/protein, 2 fat

1600 Calories:
  1 c. clam chowder
  3 oz. baked fish of choice
  baked potato
  2 T. sour cream
  vegetable salad
  2 T. fat-free salad dressing
  beverage of choice

Exchanges:
  ½ dairy, 3 bread/grain,
    1 vegetable, 0 fruit,
    3 meat/protein, 2 fat

1800 Calories:
  1 c. clam chowder
  3 oz. baked fish of choice
  baked potato
  2 T. sour cream
  vegetable salad
  2 T. fat-free salad dressing
  beverage of choice

Exchanges:
  ½ dairy, 3 bread/grain,
    1 vegetable, 0 fruit,
    3 meat/protein, 2 fat

2000 Calories:
  1 c. clam chowder
  3 oz. baked fish of choice
  baked potato
  2 T. sour cream
  vegetable salad
  2 T. fat-free salad dressing
  dinner roll
  1 t. butter
  beverage of choice

Exchanges:
  ½ dairy, 4 bread/grain,
    1 vegetable, 0 fruit,
    3 meat/protein, 3 fat

2200 Calories:
  1 c. clam chowder
  3 oz. baked fish of choice
  baked potato
  2 T. sour cream
  vegetable salad
  2 T. fat-free salad dressing
  2 dinner rolls
  1 t. butter
  beverage of choice

Exchanges:
  ½ dairy, 5 bread/grain,
    1 vegetable, 0 fruit,
    3 meat/protein, 3 fat

5

Calcium Key Cuisine
60 Recipes

Nancy's Story: Recovering from Accidental Weight Gain

Nancy, a 37-year-old nurse, was never overweight until she injured her shoulder in a car accident. Before that, she had always burned off the calories she ate. But during her recovery, which took a couple of months, she found it too stressful to watch her calories and she also stopped exercising. Her weight shot up. When she got better, she tried a couple of programs to take off the pounds, like the South Beach Diet and the Zone, but nothing worked for her. Then Nancy heard about one of our weight-loss studies and decided to participate.

She found the Calcium Key Weight-Loss Plan so much easier than the other diets she had tried. It allowed her to eat a wide range of foods, as long as she didn't overdo it on portions. And she particularly liked being allowed to have lots of dairy—the food everybody thinks is bad for dieters.

Nancy started the plan at 184 pounds, has lost 26 pounds, and is still losing. She told me she feels ecstatic about the weight loss. "I'm sure that as long as I follow the plan, I'll get back to my normal weight and never regain the weight," she said.

Welcome to the delicious, nutritious, appetite-satisfying, and easy-to-prepare recipes of *The Calcium Key*. These calorie-smart recipes are featured in the breakfasts, lunches, dinners, and snacks of the week-by-week menu plans. But you can make and enjoy them whether you choose to follow the meal plans or not.

The recipes are grouped into traditional categories like Meat, Poultry, and Egg Dishes, Soups and Casseroles. and Salads. You'll find, however, that no matter what category they're in, the recipes include (and combine in delicious ways) healthy foods like low-fat dairy, lean meat, whole grains, beans, vegetables, and fruits.

The exchange values listed in each recipe are for 1 serving. But all of the recipes (except for the blended drinks) yield 4 or more servings, so you have the choice of making the recipes for just yourself or for your family. If you're serving one or two people, just divide the recipe's ingredients— for example, if you're cooking for two, use half the amount of the ingredients of a recipe that yields 4 servings. Adjust spices to your personal flavor preferences.

Whether you prepare meals for a big family or live alone, cooking for more than one is a time-saving strategy. Freeze the uneaten portions and eat them at a later date, and spare yourself a lot of duplicated effort in the kitchen.

The recipes and meal plans were created by Tammi Hancock, R.D., a former clinical dietitian at the Mayo Clinic. Tammi has created recipes for the American Heart Association and for nearly a dozen cookbooks. She's a specialist at delicious dishes that aren't necessarily low-fat or low-carbohydrate but that reflect the proportion of macronutrients most Americans already eat: about 49% carbohydrates, 35% fat, and 16% protein. These practical recipes are part of the ease and enjoyment of The Calcium Key Weight-Loss Plan—the fact that the plan doesn't require you to make drastic and impossible-to-maintain changes in your eating habits in order to lose weight.

The recipes start with blended drinks because they're such an important and easy-to-make part of the Calcium Key Weight-Loss Plan. For recipes that include sugar or optional Splenda, calorie counts are given for sugar.

Blended Drinks

Blended drinks made with dairy and fruit—smoothies—are a wonderful way to get your dairy and fruit exchanges. They're delicious, satisfy your hunger for hours, and, if made with nonfat yogurt, are low in calories. In the meal plans, they're featured as between-meal snacks. They also make a great on-the-go breakfast, appetizer (to help you not overeat), or dessert. Kids love them.

Berry Blue Smoothie

YIELD: 1 SERVING

½ cup raspberries
½ cup blueberries
2 tablespoons grape juice concentrate

¾ cup nonfat plain yogurt
3–4 ice cubes

Combine all ingredients in a blender. Blend until smooth.

Exchanges and Nutritional Analysis:
Exchanges: 1 dairy, 2 fruit   Calcium (mg): 388   Calories: 238
% calories from carbohydrate: 77   % calories from protein: 19
% calories from fat: 4   Fiber (g): 6

Cherry Almond Smoothie

YIELD: 1 SERVING

¾ cup frozen sweet cherries
¼ teaspoon almond extract
½ tablespoon sugar or Splenda
    Granular

¾ cup nonfat plain yogurt
3–4 ice cubes

Combine all ingredients in a blender. Blend until smooth.

Exchanges and Nutritional Analysis:
Exchanges: 1 dairy, 2 fruit   Calcium (mg): 386   Calories: 223
% calories from carbohydrate: 73   % calories from protein: 22
% calories from fat: 3   Fiber (g): 3

Orange Cream Smoothie

YIELD: 1 SERVING

⅓ cup orange juice concentrate
½ teaspoon vanilla extract
1 tablespoon sugar or Splenda
    Granular

1 cup skim milk
3–4 ice cubes

Combine all ingredients in a blender. Blend until smooth.

Exchanges and Nutritional Analysis:
Exchanges: 1 dairy, 3 fruit   Calcium (mg): 332   Calories: 291
% calories from carbohydrate: 82   % calories from protein: 14
% calories from fat: 2   Fiber (g): 1

Berry Banana Smoothie

YIELD: 1 SERVING

1¼ cups fresh strawberries
½ banana
½ tablespoon sugar or Splenda
  Granular

¾ cup nonfat plain yogurt
3–4 ice cubes

Combine all ingredients in a blender. Blend until smooth.

Exchanges and Nutritional Analysis:
Exchanges: 1 dairy, 2 fruit   Calcium (mg): 395   Calories: 235
% calories from carbohydrate: 76   % calories from protein: 20
% calories from fat: 5   Fiber (g): 6

Tropical Smoothie

YIELD: 1 SERVING

¾ cup pineapple chunks
¾ cup papaya chunks
½ banana
½ tablespoon sugar or Splenda
  Granular

¾ cup nonfat plain yogurt
3–4 ice cubes

Combine all ingredients in a blender. Blend until smooth.

Exchanges and Nutritional Analysis:
Exchanges: 1 dairy, 3 fruit   Calcium (mg): 403   Calories: 279
% calories from carbohydrate: 80   % calories from protein: 17
% calories from fat: 4   Fiber (g): 5

Berry Berry Berry Smoothie

YIELD: 1 SERVING

½ cup raspberries
½ cup blueberries
¾ cup strawberries
½ tablespoon sugar or Splenda
  Granular

¾ cup nonfat plain yogurt
3–4 ice cubes

Combine all ingredients in a blender. Blend until smooth.

Exchanges and Nutritional Analysis:
Exchanges: 1 dairy, 2 fruit   Calcium (mg): 399   Calories: 230
% calories from carbohydrate: 75   % calories from protein: 20
% calories from fat: 5   Fiber (g): 9

Grape Ape Smoothie

YIELD: 1 SERVING

½ banana
3 tablespoons grape juice
   concentrate

¾ cup nonfat plain yogurt
3–4 ice cubes

Combine all ingredients in a blender. Blend until smooth.

Exchanges and Nutritional Analysis:
Exchanges: 1 dairy, 2½ fruit   Calcium (mg): 376   Calories: 254
% calories from carbohydrate: 80   % calories from protein: 18
% calories from fat: 2   Fiber (g): 2

Piña Colada Smoothie

YIELD: 1 SERVING

½ cup fresh pineapple chunks
2 teaspoons fresh lime juice
½ teaspoon coconut extract
½ tablespoon sugar or Splenda
   Granular

¾ cup nonfat plain yogurt
3–4 ice cubes

Combine all ingredients in a blender. Blend until smooth.

Exchanges and Nutritional Analysis:
Exchanges: 1 dairy, 1 fruit   Calcium (mg): 372   Calories: 174
% calories from carbohydrate: 69   % calories from protein: 24
% calories from fat: 3   Fiber (g): 1

Fuzzy Berry Smoothie

YIELD: 1 SERVING

¾ cup fresh or ½ cup drained
   canned peaches
½ cup fresh raspberries

½ tablespoon sugar
¾ cup nonfat plain yogurt
3–4 ice cubes

Combine all ingredients in a blender. Blend until smooth.

Exchanges and Nutritional Analysis:
Exchanges: 1 dairy, 2 fruit   Calcium (mg): 386   Calories: 212
% calories from carbohydrate: 75   % calories from protein: 22
% calories from fat: 3   Fiber (g): 7

Creamy Peach Smoothie

YIELD: 1 SERVING

1 cup drained canned peaches in
  juice
¼ teaspoon vanilla extract
½ tablespoon sugar or Splenda
  Granular

¾ cup nonfat plain yogurt
3–4 ice cubes

Combine all ingredients in a blender. Blend until smooth.

Exchanges and Nutritional Analysis:
Exchanges: 1 dairy, 2 fruit   Calcium (mg): 381   Calories: 239
% calories from carbohydrate: 78   % calories from protein: 19
% calories from fat: 1   Fiber (g): 3

Meat, Poultry, and Egg Dishes

These delicious dishes use healthy portions of low-fat meats and combine them with lots of low-fat dairy foods, grains, beans, and vegetables. You'll find good-for-you everyday foods like burgers and pizzas (even Pizza Burgers), an abundance of original and tasty chicken dishes, wonderful salads, a tasty quiche, and other hearty delights.

Creamy Sausage Creole

YIELD: 6 SERVINGS

2 teaspoons olive oil
⅓ cup chopped onion
1 clove garlic, minced
¼ cup chopped red bell pepper
¼ cup chopped green bell pepper
1 (14-ounce) package low-fat
  smoked sausage, cut into ¼-inch
  slices
1 (14½-ounce) can diced tomatoes,
  undrained

1 cup canned red beans, drained and
  rinsed
1 teaspoon Creole seasoning
¼ teaspoon black pepper
½ cup fat-free half-and-half
¾ cup nonfat dry milk powder
3 cups cooked brown rice

Heat olive oil in a large skillet. Add onion, garlic, and bell peppers and sauté until softened. Add sausage slices and sauté until sausage starts to brown. Stir in undrained tomatoes, beans, Creole seasoning, and black pepper. Bring to a boil and cook until most of liquid has evaporated. Combine half-and-half and dry milk powder and stir until dissolved. Add milk mixture to sausage mixture in skillet, remove from heat, and stir until combined. Serve over rice.

Exchanges and Nutritional Analysis:
Exchanges: ½ dairy, 2 bread/grain, 1 vegetable, 1 meat/protein
Calcium (mg): 169   Calories: 304   % calories from carbohydrate: 64
% calories from protein: 23   % calories from fat: 13   Fiber (g): 5

Pizza Burgers

YIELD: 6 SERVINGS

1 pound lean ground beef
1¼ cups cooked brown rice
½ cup grated Parmesan cheese
1 cup bottled or canned pizza or
  spaghetti sauce, divided
¼ teaspoon garlic powder
¼ teaspoon dried basil

¼ teaspoon dried oregano
1½ cups shredded reduced-fat
  mozzarella cheese
12 slices Italian bread
grilled onion slices and sliced black
  olives (optional)

Combine beef, rice, Parmesan cheese, ½ cup pizza sauce, garlic powder, basil, and oregano. Shape mixture into 6 oblong patties about ½ inch thick. Grill patties over medium-high heat until juices start to accumulate on top. Turn patties and cook until meat is done. Turn patties again and top each with a heaping tablespoon of remaining pizza sauce and 4 tablespoons mozzarella cheese. Place bread slices directly on grill. Grill until cheese melts and bread is lightly toasted on one side. Serve patties between toasted bread, browned sides of bread out. If desired, top burgers with grilled onion slices and black olives.

Exchanges and Nutritional Analysis:
Exchanges: 1 dairy, 2 bread/grain, 2 meat/protein
Calcium (mg): 317   Calories: 398   % calories from carbohydrate: 34
% calories from protein: 31   % calories from fat: 35   Fiber (g): 3

Reuben Pizza

YIELD: 8 SERVINGS

½ cup reduced-fat Thousand Island
  salad dressing
1 (10-ounce) prebaked pizza crust
1 cup sauerkraut, well drained

2 (2½-ounce) packages lean corned
  beef
8 ounces reduced-fat Swiss cheese,
  shredded

Spread salad dressing over pizza crust. Sprinkle sauerkraut over dressing. Arrange beef slices over sauerkraut. Sprinkle with cheese. Bake at 425 degrees for 15 minutes or until crust is browned and cheese is melted and starting to brown. Let stand 5 minutes before cutting into wedges.

Exchanges and Nutritional Analysis:
Exchanges: 1 dairy, 1 bread/grain, ½ meat/protein
Calcium (mg): 277   Calories: 227   % calories from carbohydrate: 34
% calories from protein: 29   % calories from fat: 37   Fiber (g): 1

Pork Stroganoff

YIELD: 6 SERVINGS

8 ounces dry yolk-free egg noodles
½ cup nonfat plain yogurt
½ cup nonfat dry milk powder
1 pound pork tenderloin, thinly sliced
1 teaspoon olive oil
12 ounces mushrooms, thinly sliced

¼ cup dry sherry
¼ cup beef broth
2 tablespoons flour
½ cup low-fat sour cream
½ teaspoon salt
¼ teaspoon black pepper

Prepare egg noodles according to package directions; drain. Mix yogurt and dry milk powder until smooth; set aside. Sauté pork in olive oil in a non-stick skillet; set aside. Add mushrooms to skillet and sauté until tender; add mushrooms to pork. Add sherry, broth, and flour to skillet and whisk until smooth. Bring to a boil and cook 3 to 4 minutes. Remove from heat and stir in yogurt mixture, sour cream, salt, and pepper. Add pork and mushrooms to sour cream sauce. Serve over noodles.

Exchanges and Nutritional Analysis:
Exchanges: ½ dairy, 2 bread/grain, 2 meat/protein
Calcium (mg):   159   Calories: 332   % calories from carbohydrate: 48
% calories from protein: 33   % calories from fat: 18   Fiber (g): 2

Stromboli

YIELD: 6 SERVINGS

1 (1-pound) loaf frozen bread dough
1 egg
1 tablespoon olive oil
1–2 tablespoons chopped basil
½ teaspoon garlic powder
½ teaspoon black pepper
¼ teaspoon salt

4 ounces low-fat ham, thinly sliced
⅔ cup frozen Italian sausage-style
   vegetable protein crumbles
1½ cups shredded reduced-fat
   mozzarella cheese
½ cup grated Parmesan cheese,
   divided

Place frozen dough on a greased plate and cover with greased plastic wrap. Set aside in a warm, draft-free place and allow to rise for 4 hours or until doubled in size. Roll out dough on a floured surface into a 10 × 12–inch rectangle. Beat together egg, olive oil, basil, garlic powder, black pepper, and salt in a small bowl. Spread about half of egg mixture over dough. Arrange ham on dough, leaving a 1-inch border around the sides. Sprinkle sausage crumbles over ham and top with mozzarella cheese and ¼ cup Parmesan cheese. Drizzle remaining egg mixture over cheese. Roll up dough jelly-roll fashion, starting with the long end. Seal seam and tuck ends under roll. Place roll seam-side down on a baking sheet. Sprinkle remaining ¼ cup Parmesan cheese on top. Bake at 350 degrees for 30 minutes or until browned. Remove from oven and let stand 5 minutes before slicing.

Exchanges and Nutritional Analysis:
Exchanges: 1 dairy, 2 bread/grain, 1 meat/protein
Calcium (mg): 304   Calories: 372   % calories from carbohydrate: 43
% calories from protein: 23   % calories from fat: 33   Fiber (g): 2

Stuffed Chicken Popovers

YIELD: 6 SERVINGS

Popovers:
1 egg
2 egg whites
1 cup skim milk

1 cup all-purpose flour
½ teaspoon salt

Filling:
1 tablespoon all-purpose flour
½ cup skim milk
1 cup shredded reduced-fat cheddar
    cheese
½ cup shredded American cheese

2 cups broccoli florets
1 pound chicken breast tenders, each
    cut in half lengthwise
¼ teaspoon garlic salt or seasoned
    salt

To make the popovers, lightly beat egg and egg whites in a medium bowl. Mix in milk. Add flour and salt and mix just until batter is smooth. Divide batter among 6 regular-size muffin cups, being careful not to overfill cups. Bake at 450 degrees for 20 minutes. Decrease oven temperature to 350 degrees and bake 15 minutes longer or until browned.

Meanwhile, prepare filling. Whisk flour and milk together in a saucepan until smooth. Cook and stir over medium heat until mixture thickens. Add cheeses and stir until melted and smooth. Cook broccoli with a small amount of water in the microwave on high power for 2 minutes or until tender. Drain broccoli and add to cheese sauce. Cover to keep warm. Season chicken breast tenders with garlic salt and sauté in a nonstick skillet until done.

Immediately after baking, remove popovers from oven and place on individual serving plates. Break into top of popovers. Stuff chicken into popovers. Top with broccoli cheese sauce.

Exchanges and Nutritional Analysis:
Exchanges: 1 dairy, 1 bread/grain, 2 meat/protein
Calcium (mg): 332   Calories: 299   % calories from carbohydrate: 30
% calories from protein: 44   % calories from fat: 26   Fiber (g): 1

Greek Couscous Salad

YIELD: 6 SERVINGS

1⅓ cups water
1 cup dry couscous
1 pound boneless, skinless chicken breast, cooked and diced
6 ounces crumbled feta cheese
¼ cup Parmesan cheese
10 black olives, sliced

¼ cup dried cranberries
2 cups chopped cucumber
2 tablespoons olive oil
¼ cup red wine vinegar
2 tablespoons lemon juice
1 teaspoon salt
2 teaspoons dried oregano

Bring water to a boil in a saucepan. Stir in couscous, remove from heat, and cover. Let stand 5 minutes. Transfer cooked couscous to a mixing bowl and cool. Add chicken, feta and Parmesan cheeses, olive slices, cranberries, and cucumber to mixing bowl. In a small bowl, whisk together olive oil, vinegar, lemon juice, salt, and oregano. Pour dressing over couscous mixture. Toss until well mixed.

Exchanges and Nutritional Analysis:
Exchanges: ½ dairy, 2 bread/grain, 2 meat/protein
Calcium (mg): 220   Calories: 379   % calories from carbohydrate: 37
% calories from protein: 30   % calories from fat: 33   Fiber (g): 2

Asian Chicken Salad

YIELD: 4 SERVINGS

½ cup nonfat plain yogurt
½ cup nonfat dry milk powder
1 tablespoon Splenda Granular (optional)
1 tablespoon soy sauce
6 cups mixed salad greens
⅓ cup raw pea pods, cut into thirds

1½ cups cooked chopped chicken
1 (11-ounce) can mandarin oranges in light syrup, drained
1 (8-ounce) can sliced water chestnuts, drained and julienned
½ cup canned rice noodles

Combine yogurt, milk powder, and soy sauce in a small bowl. Mix well until smooth; set aside. In a large salad bowl, combine greens, pea pods, chicken, oranges, and water chestnuts. Pour yogurt dressing over salad. Toss until mixed. Sprinkle rice noodles on top just before serving.

Exchanges and Nutritional Analysis:
Exchanges: ½ dairy, ½ bread/grain, ½ fruit, 1 vegetable, 2 meat/protein
Calcium (mg): 234   Calories: 220   % calories from carbohydrate: 47
% calories from protein: 40   % calories from fat: 12   Fiber (g): 5

Chicken Cheese Steak
YIELD: 4 SERVINGS

½ cup sliced onion
2 teaspoons olive oil, divided
6 ounces mushrooms, sliced
½ pound chicken tenders, quartered lengthwise

½ teaspoon seasoned salt
1 (8-ounce) loaf multigrain French bread
4 ounces reduced-fat Swiss cheese
¼ cup sliced roasted red peppers

Sauté onion in 1 teaspoon olive oil until softened in a nonstick skillet. Add mushrooms and sauté until softened. Remove vegetables from skillet and keep warm. Add remaining teaspoon of olive oil to skillet over medium-high heat. Sprinkle chicken with seasoned salt and add to skillet. Sauté until chicken is done. Cut French bread in half lengthwise. Add sautéed chicken to bread. Cover with cheese. Spoon sautéed vegetables and roasted red peppers on top. Cut into 4 pieces and serve.

Exchanges and Nutritional Analysis:
Exchanges: 1 dairy, 2 bread/grain, 2 meat/protein
Calcium (mg): 281   Calories: 353   % calories from carbohydrate: 43
% calories from protein: 35   % calories from fat: 22   Fiber (g): 4

Stuffed Chicken with Creamy Pesto Sauce
YIELD: 4 SERVINGS

4 (4-ounce) boneless, skinless chicken breasts
4 (½-ounce) slices skim milk mozzarella cheese
½ cup grated Parmesan cheese, divided

2 tablespoons dry bread crumbs
2 small cloves garlic
½ teaspoon salt
2 cups packed basil leaves
¼ teaspoon black pepper
6 tablespoons fat-free half-and-half

Place chicken breasts, boned-side down, on a flat surface. Cut a slit in the top of each breast, cutting about halfway into the meat; be careful not to cut too deep. From inside the slit, cut breast horizontally on both sides, forming a pocket; again, be careful not to cut through to the bottom of the breast—holes in the bottom of the breast will allow cheese to escape while baking. Place a mozzarella cheese slice in the pocket of each breast, folding meat over the top to enclose the cheese. Combine 2 tablespoons Parmesan cheese and bread crumbs in a shallow dish. Lightly coat chicken breasts with crumb mixture and place cut-side up on a wire rack over a baking sheet. Bake at 450 degrees for 15 to 20 minutes or until chicken is done.

Meanwhile, prepare pesto. Mash garlic with salt and combine with basil, pepper, remaining 6 tablespoons Parmesan cheese, and 2 tablespoons half-and-half in a food processor. Process until basil is finely chopped. Spoon mixture into a saucepan. Add remaining 4 tablespoons half-and-half. Cook, stirring occasionally, for about 5 minutes; do not boil. To serve, drizzle sauce in a circle on individual serving plates. Place a chicken breast in the center of each circle.

Exchanges and Nutritional Analysis:
Exchanges: 1 dairy, 3 meat/protein   Calcium (mg): 315   Calories: 243
% calories from carbohydrate: 13   % calories from protein: 61
% calories from fat: 26   Fiber (g): 1

Caesar Tortellini Salad

YIELD: 8 SERVINGS

1¼ pounds boneless, skinless chicken breast
1 (19-ounce) package frozen cheese tortellini
¾ cup reduced-fat Caesar salad dressing
1 cup grated Parmesan cheese, divided
¾ teaspoon black pepper
8 cups chopped Romaine lettuce
½ cup grape or cherry tomato halves

Cook chicken on a grill over medium-high heat until done. Cool completely, then cut into cubes or long, thin strips. Cook cheese tortellini according to package instructions; drain and cool. Combine chicken and tortellini. Add dressing and toss until mixed. Add ¾ cup cheese and pepper and toss to mix. Place lettuce in a large salad bowl or divide among individual salad plates. Spoon tortellini mixture on top. Sprinkle with remaining cheese. Top with tomatoes.

Exchanges and Nutritional Analysis:
Exchanges: 1 dairy, 1½ bread/grain, 1 vegetable, 2 meat/protein
Calcium (mg): 291   Calories: 342   % calories from carbohydrate: 42
% calories from protein: 36   % calories from fat: 22   Fiber (g): 3

Chicken Enchiladas in White Cream Sauce

YIELD: 8 SERVINGS

½ cup sliced green onions
2 cloves chopped garlic
2 teaspoons olive oil
3 cups cooked chopped chicken
2 cups fat-free chicken broth
2 tablespoons cornstarch
2 cups shredded reduced-fat
  Monterey Jack cheese, divided
3 tablespoons light mayonnaise-type
  salad dressing

⅓ cup plain nonfat yogurt
1 (4-ounce) can chopped green
  chilies
1 (2¼-ounce) can sliced black
  olives, drained
8 (8-inch) flour tortillas
salsa (optional)

In a medium skillet, sauté onions and garlic in olive oil until softened. Add chicken and continue to cook and stir until heated through. Set aside. Pour chicken broth in a saucepan. Mix in cornstarch until smooth. Bring to a boil. Cook and stir 2 minutes. Add ¾ cup cheese, salad dressing, yogurt, chilies, and olives. Stir until smooth. Add ¾ cup of cheese sauce to chicken mixture. Fill tortillas with chicken mixture, placing about ⅓ cup of mixture across center of each tortilla. Roll tortillas and place in a greased 9 × 13–inch pan, seam-side down. Pour remainder of sauce over tortillas. Top with remaining cheese. Cover lightly with foil and bake at 350 degrees for 25 minutes or until sauce is bubbly. Uncover and cook another 10 to 15 minutes or until cheese is just starting to brown. Serve with salsa.

Exchanges and Nutritional Analysis:
Exchanges: 1 dairy, 1 bread/grain, 2 meat/protein
Calcium (mg): 34   Calories: 344   % calories from carbohydrate: 35
% calories from protein: 36   % calories from fat: 29   Fiber (g): 3

Turkey Tet-rotini

YIELD: 6 SERVINGS

3 cups sliced mushrooms (about 6
  ounces)
⅓ cup chopped red bell pepper
2 teaspoons olive oil
2 cups cooked chopped chicken
12 ounces dry tricolored rotini,
  cooked and drained
⅓ cup flour
1 cup chicken broth

1 cup skim milk
1 cup dry milk powder
½ cup shredded cheddar cheese
½ cup shredded Swiss cheese
3 tablespoons dry sherry
½ teaspoon salt
¼ teaspoon black pepper
¼ cup grated Parmesan cheese

Sauté mushrooms and red bell pepper in olive oil in a nonstick skillet until softened; transfer to a large mixing bowl. Add chicken and cooked rotini to bowl and set aside. Add flour and chicken broth to skillet and whisk until flour is dissolved. Bring mixture to a boil, stirring frequently. Add milk and milk powder, and cook and stir until hot. Stir in cheddar and Swiss cheeses, sherry, salt, and pepper. Cook and stir until cheese is melted. Pour cheese sauce over chicken and rotini in mixing bowl. Mix well and transfer to a 2-quart baking dish. Sprinkle Parmesan cheese on top. Bake, covered, at 350 degrees for 50 minutes or until hot.

Exchanges and Nutritional Analysis:
Exchanges: 1½ dairy, 2 bread/grain, 2 meat/protein
Calcium (mg): 442　Calories: 433　% calories from carbohydrate: 48
% calories from protein: 30　% calories from fat: 21　Fiber (g): 2

Hashbrown Quiche

YIELD: 6 SERVINGS

3 cups refrigerated hash brown
　potatoes
½ cup chopped onion
2 teaspoons butter
2 ounces lean Canadian bacon, diced
2 eggs
3 egg whites
1 cup skim milk
½ teaspoon salt

½ teaspoon black pepper
½ (10-ounce) package frozen
　chopped spinach, thawed and
　squeezed dry
¾ cup shredded reduced-fat cheddar
　cheese
¾ cup shredded reduced-fat Swiss
　cheese

Sauté potatoes and onion in butter in a nonstick skillet until potatoes turn golden brown. Pat hash browns into a greased 9-inch pie pan to form a crust. Add Canadian bacon to skillet and sauté briefly; set aside. Beat eggs and egg whites with milk, salt, and pepper in a mixing bowl. Add sautéed bacon, spinach, and cheeses. Mix well and pour over hash browns in pie pan. Bake at 375 degrees for 45 minutes or until center is set. Let stand 10 minutes before serving.

Exchanges and Nutritional Analysis:
Exchanges: 1 dairy, ½ bread/grain, 1 meat/protein
Calcium (mg): 368　Calories: 239　% calories from carbohydrate: 35
% calories from protein: 30　% calories from fat: 35　Fiber (g): 2

Fish and Seafood

Here's a healthy bounty from the sea, combined with delicious dairy-based dressings and sauces.

Grilled Fish Tacos

YIELD: 8 SERVINGS

1½ pounds swordfish steaks
2 tablespoons lime juice
1 clove chopped garlic
½ cup nonfat plain yogurt
2 tablespoons cider vinegar
½ teaspoon salt
4 cups shredded cabbage or coleslaw mix

4 green onions, tops only, sliced
¼ cup chopped cilantro
2 cups shredded reduced-fat Monterey Jack cheese
8 (8-inch) flour tortillas

Place fish in a plastic resealable bag with lime juice and garlic. Marinate fish 15 to 30 minutes. In a small bowl, combine yogurt, vinegar, and salt. Place cabbage, onions, and cilantro in a separate bowl. Pour yogurt dressing on top and toss until well coated. Grill fish over medium-high heat, turning once, for 5 to 10 minutes or until meat flakes easily. Break fish into chunks or slice. To assemble tacos, spoon cabbage mixture onto flour tortillas. Top with fish and cheese. Fold tortillas to enclose filling.

Exchanges and Nutritional Analysis:
Exchanges: 1 dairy, 1 bread/grain, 2 meat/protein
Calcium (mg): 317   Calories: 318   % calories from carbohydrate: 36
% calories from protein: 38   % calories from fat: 26   Fiber (g): 3

Tuna Cheese Salad

YIELD: 4 SERVINGS

1 (7.1-ounce) foil package tuna
6 ounces dry shell macaroni, cooked and drained
¾ cup diced reduced-fat Monterey Jack cheese
½ cup sliced green onion
¼ cup chopped red bell pepper

¼ cup finely chopped celery
¼ teaspoon salt
¼ teaspoon black pepper
½ teaspoon celery salt
1¼ cups low-fat cottage cheese
¼ cup nonfat plain yogurt
8 cherry tomatoes, halved

Combine tuna, cooked macaroni, Monterey Jack cheese, onion, bell pepper, celery, salt, pepper, and celery salt in a bowl. Blend cottage cheese and yogurt in a food processor or blender until smooth. Add cottage cheese mixture to salad and toss until mixed. Garnish salad with cherry tomato halves.

Exchanges and Nutritional Analysis:
Exchanges: 1 dairy, 2 bread/grain, 2 meat/protein
Calcium (mg): 287   Calories: 345   % calories from carbohydrate: 45
% calories from protein: 39   % calories from fat: 16   Fiber (g): 2

Parmesan Roughy
YIELD: 4 SERVINGS

½ cup grated Parmesan cheese
½ cup soft bread crumbs (about 1 slice)
½ teaspoon lemon pepper

¼ teaspoon garlic powder
½ cup nonfat plain yogurt
¼ cup skim milk
1 pound orange roughy fillets

Combine cheese, bread crumbs, lemon pepper, and garlic powder in a shallow dish. In a separate dish, combine yogurt and milk. Pat fish fillets dry with paper towels. Dip fillets in yogurt mixture, then roll in bread crumb mixture until well coated. Place breaded fillets on a wire rack on a baking sheet. Bake at 425 degrees for 20 minutes or until fish flakes easily when tested with a fork.

Exchanges and Nutritional Analysis:
Exchanges: 1 dairy, 2½ meat/protein   Calcium (mg): 257
Calories: 169   % calories from carbohydrate: 20
% calories from protein: 58   % calories from fat: 22   Fiber (g): 1

Pita Shrimp
YIELD: 4 SERVINGS

1 (4-ounce) package frozen cooked shrimp, thawed, chopped, and drained
2 tablespoons low-fat mayonnaise
2 tablespoons nonfat plain yogurt
½ teaspoon lemon juice

¼ teaspoon seafood seasoning blend
2 egg whites
4 ounces Edam cheese, shredded
4 teaspoons butter, softened
4 (6-inch) pita bread

Combine shrimp, mayonnaise, yogurt, lemon juice, and seafood seasoning. Beat egg whites until stiff. Fold cheese into egg whites. Spread butter over one side of each pita. Spoon shrimp mixture over butter on pita. Spread cheese mixture over shrimp. Place on a baking sheet. Bake at 400 degrees for 20 minutes or until cheese and crust are golden brown. Cut into quarters and serve immediately.

Exchanges and Nutritional Analysis:
Exchanges: 1 dairy, 1½ bread/grain, 1meat/protein, ½ fat
Calcium (mg): 245   Calories: 360   % calories from carbohydrate: 38
% calories from protein: 23   % calories from fat: 39   Fiber (g): 4

Grain Dishes and Breads

This section specializes in good-for-you grains. You'll find a delicious risotto, cornbread, muffins that are marvelous as a breakfast meal (check out Tammi's Minnesota Muffins, named after our recipe developer, who says her kids love them in their lunch boxes), and a French toast that delivers plenty of mouthwatering taste for only 251 calories per serving.

Creamy Spring Risotto
YIELD: 4 SERVINGS

½ cup chopped onion
1 carrot, julienned
2 teaspoons olive oil
1 cup dry arborio rice
2 cups fat-free chicken broth

1 cup evaporated milk
1 bunch asparagus, ends trimmed,
  cut into 1-inch pieces
1 zucchini, julienned
¼ cup grated Parmesan cheese

Sauté onion and carrot in olive oil until softened. Add rice and sauté briefly. Add chicken broth, ½ cup at a time, cooking and stirring between additions until all broth is absorbed before adding more. After all broth is absorbed, stir in milk, asparagus, and zucchini. Cook and stir until milk is absorbed and vegetables are tender. Mix in cheese.

Exchanges and Nutritional Analysis:
Exchanges: 1 dairy, 2 bread/grain, 3 vegetable
Calcium (mg): 299   Calories: 358   % calories from carbohydrate: 68
% calories from protein: 19   % calories from fat: 13   Fiber (g): 5

Mexican Cornbread

YIELD: 9 SERVINGS

½ cup cornmeal
1 cup all-purpose flour
1 tablespoon baking powder
½ teaspoon salt
1 egg
2 egg whites
½ cup nonfat dry milk powder

1 cup skim milk
1 tablespoon canola oil
1 jalapeño pepper, chopped
3 tablespoons chopped red bell pepper
1½ cups shredded reduced-fat Colby-Jack cheese

Combine cornmeal, flour, baking powder, and salt in a mixing bowl. In a separate bowl, beat egg and egg whites. Dissolve milk powder in milk. Add milk mixture and oil to eggs and mix. Add mixture to dry ingredients and blend until smooth. Stir in jalapeño and bell peppers and cheese. Pour batter into a nonstick 9 × 9–inch square baking pan. Bake at 350 degrees for 40 minutes. Cool slightly and cut into squares.

Exchanges and Nutritional Analysis:
Exchanges: 1 dairy, 1 bread/grain   Calcium (mg): 309
Calories: 185   % calories from carbohydrate: 48
% calories from protein: 23   % calories from fat: 29   Fiber (g): 1

Ham and Cheese Muffins

YIELD: 12 SERVINGS

1½ cups all-purpose flour
½ cup cornmeal
1 tablespoons Splenda Granular
1 tablespoon baking powder
½ teaspoon salt
½ cup shredded reduced-fat cheddar cheese

4 ounces lean ham or Canadian bacon, finely diced
2 egg whites
1 cup milk
½ cup low-fat cottage cheese
2 tablespoons vegetable oil
salsa (optional)

Combine flour, cornmeal, Splenda, baking powder, and salt in a large bowl; mix well. Stir in cheese and ham. In a separate bowl, beat egg whites. Mix in milk, cottage cheese, and oil. Add milk mixture to dry ingredients and stir until just moistened. Spoon batter into nonstick muffin cups. Bake at 400 degrees for 20 to 25 minutes or until golden brown. Serve with salsa on the side.

Exchanges and Nutritional Analysis:
Exchanges: ½ dairy, 1 bread/grain   Calcium (mg): 145
Calories: 142   % calories from carbohydrate: 52
% calories from protein: 22   % calories from fat: 26   Fiber (g): 1

Tammi's Minnesota Muffins

YIELD: 12 MUFFINS

1 cup all-purpose flour
1/2 cup cornmeal
1/3 cup Splenda Granular
1/2 teaspoon salt
1 tablespoon baking powder
3/4 cup cold cooked wild rice

1 egg
3/4 cup skim milk
2/3 cup nonfat dry milk powder
1/4 cup vegetable oil
1 cup blueberries

Combine flour, cornmeal, Splenda, salt, and baking powder in a large bowl; mix well. Stir in wild rice. In a separate bowl, beat egg. Mix in milk, milk powder, and oil until smooth. Add milk mixture to dry ingredients and stir until just moistened. Fold in blueberries. Spoon batter into nonstick muffin cups. Bake at 400 degrees for 15 to 20 minutes or until golden brown.

Exchanges and Nutritional Analysis:
Exchanges: 1/2 dairy, 1 bread/grain   Calcium (mg): 138
Calories: 146   % calories from carbohydrate: 55
% calories from protein: 12   % calories from fat: 33   Fiber (g): 1

Baked French Toast with Maple Yogurt and Fruit

YIELD: 6 SERVINGS

6 slices 1-inch thick bread (or
  Texas Toast)
1 egg
4 egg whites
1 cup dry milk powder
1 1/4 cups milk
1/2 teaspoon vanilla

1/8 teaspoon cinnamon
1/2 cup nonfat plain yogurt
3 tablespoons maple syrup
3 cups mixed berries, such as sliced
  strawberries, blueberries, and
  raspberries

Arrange bread in a greased 9 × 13–inch glass baking dish; set aside. Beat egg and egg whites in a mixing bowl. Dissolve dry milk powder in milk. Add milk mixture, vanilla, and cinnamon to eggs and mix well. Pour mixture slowly over bread in dish. Bake at 350 degrees for 25 minutes or until bread is golden brown. Meanwhile, mix yogurt and syrup in a small bowl. Spoon yogurt mixture over individual servings of baked French toast. Top with fresh berries.

Exchanges and Nutritional Analysis:
Exchanges: 1 dairy, 1 bread/grain, 1 fruit, 1/2 meat/protein
Calcium (mg): 286   Calories: 251   % calories from carbohydrate: 69
% calories from protein: 22   % calories from fat: 9   Fiber (g): 4

Soups and Casseroles

Soups are an important part of the Calcium Key Weight-Loss Plan. Scientific studies show that starting a meal with soup—or making a meal of soup—is a great way to feel full on fewer calories, speeding weight loss. In this section, you'll find a variety of tasty variations on classic soups, all of which are great as a meal.

Cheese Tortellini Soup

YIELD: 8 SERVINGS

1 cup chopped onion
2 cloves garlic, pressed
1 teaspoon olive oil
1 (49-ounce) can fat-free chicken broth
1 tablespoon chicken soup base
2 cups cooked chopped chicken
1 cup chopped carrot
1/2 teaspoon dried basil

1/2 teaspoon dried oregano
1 (16-ounce) package frozen cheese tortellini
1 (10-ounce) package frozen chopped broccoli
1 cup fat-free half-and-half
1/4 cup cornstarch
2/3 cup nonfat dry milk powder
1/2 cup Parmesan cheese

Sauté onion and garlic in olive oil until softened but not browned. Add broth, soup base, chicken, carrot, basil, and oregano. Bring to a boil. Reduce heat and simmer until carrot is tender. Stir in tortellini and broccoli. In a small bowl, mix half-and-half with cornstarch smooth. Stir in dry milk powder until dissolved. Add milk mixture to soup and stir to blend. Cook, stirring frequently, until mixture is thickened. Top each serving with 1 tablespoon Parmesan cheese.

Exchanges and Nutritional Analysis:
Exchanges: 1 dairy, 2 bread/grain, 1 meat/protein   Calcium (mg): 315
Calories: 340   % calories from carbohydrate: 50
% calories from fat: 20   % calories from protein: 30   Fiber (g): 3

Mediterranean Lentil Soup

YIELD: 6 (1 1/3-CUP) SERVINGS

1/2 cup finely chopped celery
1/2 cup finely chopped carrot

1/2 cup chopped onion
1 clove garlic, minced

2 teaspoons olive oil
1½ cups dry lentils (about 8 ounces), sorted and rinsed
3 (14-ounce) cans fat-free chicken broth
¼ teaspoon dried thyme, crushed
1 bay leaf
¼ teaspoon ground cumin
¼ teaspoon salt

¼ teaspoon black pepper
1 cup frozen Italian sausage-style vegetable protein crumbles
1 (14½-ounce) can diced tomatoes, undrained
2 tablespoons dry brown rice
½ cup dry white wine
2 cups shredded reduced-fat mozzarella cheese

Sauté celery, carrot, onion, and garlic in olive oil in a 3-quart saucepan until softened. Add lentils, broth, thyme, bay leaf, cumin, salt, and pepper and bring to a boil. Reduce heat, cover, and simmer about 20 minutes. Stir in vegetable protein crumbles, tomatoes, rice, and wine. Bring to a boil. Reduce heat, cover, and simmer 25 minutes or until lentils are tender. Remove bay leaf. Top each serving with ⅓ cup cheese.

Exchanges and Nutritional Analysis:
Exchanges: 1 dairy, 1½ bread/grain, 1 vegetable, 2 meat/protein
Calcium (mg): 299   Calories: 364   % calories from carbohydrate: 43
% calories from protein: 32   % calories from fat: 22   Fiber (g): 17

Wild Rice Soup

YIELD: 6 SERVINGS

¾ cup dry wild rice
1½ cup water
1 tablespoon butter
1 cup chopped mushrooms
½ cup chopped onion
½ cup chopped celery
1 cup julienned carrot
¼ cup flour

4 cups fat-free chicken broth
1½ cups dry milk powder
1 cup milk
1 cup cooked chopped chicken
1 tablespoon chicken base
2 tablespoons cornstarch
2 tablespoons water

Combine rice and water in a large saucepan and bring to a boil. Reduce heat to a simmer, cover, and cook 40 minutes or until tender; drain and set aside. Melt butter in saucepan. Add mushrooms, onion, celery, and carrot and sauté until vegetables are softened but not browned. Add flour and toss to coat vegetables. Whisk in broth until flour is dissolved. Bring mixture to a boil. Reduce heat and simmer soup 2 to 3 minutes. Dissolve milk powder in milk. Add milk mixture, chicken, and soup base to soup. Cook until heated. If a thicker soup is desired, dissolve cornstarch in water and stir into soup. Cook until thickened.

Exchanges and Nutritional Analysis:
Exchanges: 1 dairy, 1 bread/grain, 1 vegetable, 1 meat/protein
Calcium (mg): 281   Calories: 271   % calories from carbohydrate: 56
% calories from protein: 29   % calories from fat: 15   Fiber (g): 3

Chicken Enchilada Soup

YIELD: 10 SERVINGS

1 (16-ounce) package dried navy beans
½ tablespoon vegetable oil
1 cup chopped onion
2 cloves garlic, minced
1 teaspoon ground cumin
1 (28-ounce) can tomatoes, drained
2 (14½-ounce) cans fat-free chicken broth

1 (8-ounce) can tomato sauce
2 (4-ounce) cans chopped green chilies
½ cup chopped cilantro
2 teaspoons dried oregano
2 cups cooked chopped chicken
2 cup shredded reduced-fat Colby-Jack cheese, divided
10 thin corn tortillas

Soak beans according to package directions. Drain and rinse beans. Heat oil in a 6-quart pot. Add onion, garlic, and cumin and sauté until onion is softened but not browned. Add drained beans, drained tomatoes, and broth. Puree mixture with a hand blender, or puree in batches in a food processor. Stir in tomato sauce, chilies, cilantro, oregano, and chicken. Heat to a boil. Reduce heat and cover. Simmer on low heat for 1 hour or more, stirring occasionally. When ready to serve, stir in 1 cup cheese until melted. Serve remaining 1 cup cheese and tortilla strips on the side as soup toppings. To make tortilla strips, stack tortillas and cut in half. Cut each half-stack into thin strips. Spread strips on a baking sheet. Bake at 350 degrees, tossing frequently, for 15 minutes or until crispy and starting to lightly brown.

Exchanges and Nutritional Analysis:
Exchanges: ½ dairy, 2 bread/grain, 1 vegetable, 2 meat/protein
Calcium (mg): 343   Calories: 353   % calories from carbohydrate: 48
% calories from protein: 30   % calories from fat: 22   Fiber (g): 14

Seafood Chowder

YIELD: 6 SERVINGS

2 slices bacon
1 cup chopped onion
1 pound russet potatoes, peeled and diced
¼ teaspoon salt
¼ teaspoon pepper
2 cups fish stock, or fish bouillon to equal 2 cups
1 (8-ounce) cod fillet, cut into chunks

4 ounces medium-size shrimp, peeled, deveined, and halved
4 ounces sea scallops, each cut into 3 or 4 pieces
2 tablespoons chopped parsley
½ tablespoon chopped chives
1 cup fat-free half-and-half
1⅓ cups nonfat dry milk powder
2 tablespoons cornstarch

Cook bacon in a large saucepan over medium-low heat to render fat. Set bacon aside, leaving fat in saucepan. Add onion and potato to bacon fat and sauté over medium heat until softened but not browned. Season with salt and pepper. Add fish stock and bring to a boil. Add cod, shrimp, scallops, parsley, and chives. Bring to a simmer and cook 4 to 5 minutes or until seafood is done. In small bowl, combine half-and-half, dry milk powder and cornstarch and stir until smooth. Add milk mixture to soup and cook, stirring often, until mixture is thickened; do not boil. Reduce heat to low and cook 10 to 15 minutes. Crumble cooked bacon and sprinkle on top individual servings.

Exchanges and Nutritional Analysis:
Exchanges: 1 dairy, 1 bread/grain, 2 meat/protein   Calcium (mg): 271
Calories: 226   % calories from carbohydrate: 53
% calories from protein: 40   % calories from fat: 7   Fiber (g): 2

Baked Potato Soup

YIELD: 6 SERVINGS

1½ pounds russet potatoes
½ tablespoon butter
½ cup chopped onion
⅓ cup all-purpose flour
½ teaspoon salt
½ teaspoon black pepper
½ teaspoon seasoned salt
1 (14½-ounce) can fat-free chicken broth

⅔ cup nonfat dry milk powder
2 cups skim milk
1½ cups reduced-fat cheddar cheese, divided
½ cup fat-free sour cream
2 slices bacon, cooked and crumbled
chopped fresh chives

Bake potatoes in oven or microwave until tender. When cool enough to handle, peel potatoes. Mash half of the potatoes and dice the other half; set aside. Melt butter in a large saucepan. Add onion and sauté until tender but not browned. Add flour, salt, pepper and seasoned salt and stir to coat onions. Whisk in chicken broth until flour is dissolved. Bring to a boil, stirring frequently. Reduce heat to a simmer and cook and stir until thickened. Dissolve milk powder in skim milk. Add milk mixture and mashed and diced potatoes to soup. Cook until soup is heated. Stir in 1 cup cheese and cook and stir until melted. Add sour cream and stir until blended. Cook until heated. Top individual servings with a rounded tablespoon of remaining cheese and a sprinkle of bacon and chives.

Exchanges and Nutritional Analysis:
Exchanges: 1½ dairy, 1 bread/grain, ½ fat   Calcium (mg): 496
Calories: 293   % calories from carbohydrate: 51
% calories from protein: 27   % calories from fat: 22   Fiber (g): 3

Chili Cheese Casserole
YIELD: 6 SERVINGS

1 egg
4 egg whites
1 cup milk
1 cup low-fat cottage cheese
½ teaspoon salt
1 (4-ounce) can chopped chilis
1 (15-ounce) can black beans, rinsed and drained

2 tablespoons chopped red bell pepper
¼ cup sliced green onion, divided
10 (6-inch) corn tortillas, cut in half or quarters
1½ cups reduced-fat Colby-Jack cheese

Whisk together egg, egg whites, milk, cottage cheese, and salt. In a separate bowl, combine chilies, beans, bell pepper, and 2 tablespoons green onion. In a greased 2-quart casserole dish, layer casserole as follows: one-third of tortilla pieces, half of cottage cheese, one-third of Colby-Jack cheese, half of bean mixture, one-third tortilla pieces, remaining cottage cheese, one-third of Colby-Jack cheese, remaining bean mixture, remaining tortilla pieces, and remaining Colby-Jack cheese. Sprinkle remaining 2 tablespoons green onion on top. Bake at 375 degrees for 45 minutes or until eggs are set and a knife inserted in the center comes out clean.

Exchanges and Nutritional Analysis:
Exchanges: 1 dairy, 1 bread/grain, 1 meat/protein   Calcium (mg): 447
Calories: 264   % calories from carbohydrate: 38
% calories from protein: 35   % calories from fat: 26   Fiber (g): 6

Melon Berry Soup

YIELD: 6 SERVINGS

1 quart strawberries, hulled
1 cup orange juice
2 tablespoons quick-cooking tapioca
½ teaspoon lemon zest
¼ cup Splenda Granular

¼ honeydew melon, peeled and cut
    into chunks
1 cup nonfat dry milk powder
2 cups buttermilk

Puree strawberries with orange juice in a blender. Transfer pureed mixture to a saucepan. Cook over medium heat until hot. Place tapioca in a small bowl. Add a small amount of heated strawberry mixture to tapioca and stir until dissolved. Add dissolved mixture back to saucepan and stir until blended. Add lemon zest and sugar and bring to a boil. Cook and stir for 2 minutes. Remove from heat and stir in Splenda. Puree melon with milk. Dissolve milk powder in buttermilk mixture in a blender until smooth. Add melon mixture to soup. Stir until combined. Refrigerate until chilled. Serve cold.

Exchanges and Nutritional Analysis:
Exchanges: 1 dairy, 1 fruit   Calcium (mg): 256   Calories: 211
% calories from carbohydrate: 81   % calories from protein: 14
% calories from fat: 5   Fiber (g): 3

Salads

Some of the vegetable-packed salads in this section are quick-and-easy meals rather than side dishes or appetizers.

Apple Carrot Salad

YIELD: 8 SERVINGS

1 large Granny Smith apple,
    unpeeled and chopped
1 teaspoon lemon juice
3 carrots, shredded
1 cup halved red seedless grapes

2 tablespoons chopped walnuts
¾ cup nonfat plain yogurt
2 tablespoons orange juice
    concentrate

In a medium bowl, toss apple with lemon juice to prevent browning. Add carrot, grapes and walnuts and mix. In a separate container, combine yogurt and orange juice concentrate. Mix. Pour yogurt mixture over salad and toss until combined.

Exchanges and Nutritional Analysis:
Exchanges: ½ dairy, 1 fruit, 1 vegetable   Calcium (mg): 121
Calories: 151   % calories from carbohydrate: 73
% calories from protein: 11   % calories from fat: 15   Fiber (g): 4

Chef's Pasta Salad

YIELD: 4 SERVINGS

¾ cup dry whole-wheat spiral macaroni, cooked al dente and drained
3 ounces reduced-fat cheddar
cheese, diced
3 ounces reduced-fat Swiss cheese,
diced
2 ounces low-fat ham, cut into strips

2 ounces deli turkey, cut into strips
⅓ cup reduced-fat Italian salad
dressing
6 cups chopped leafy lettuce
1 hard-cooked egg, chopped
8 cherry tomatoes, halved

Combine drained pasta, cheeses, ham, and turkey in a mixing bowl. Pour dressing over top and toss. Place lettuce in a serving bowl. Spoon pasta mixture on top. Sprinkle with egg and garnish with tomatoes.

Exchanges and Nutritional Analysis:
Exchanges: 1½ dairy, ½ bread/grain, 1 meat/poultry   Calcium (mg): 472
Calories: 273   % calories from carbohydrate: 32
% calories from protein: 34   % calories from fat: 34   Fiber (g): 4

Fruit and Cheese Salad

YIELD: 6 SERVINGS

1½ cups chopped red pear
1½ cups chopped Granny Smith
apple
1 cup seedless grapes, halved
6 ounces reduced-fat cheddar
cheese, diced

¼ cup chopped walnuts
1½ tablespoons orange juice
concentrate
1 tablespoon olive oil

Combine pear, apple, grapes, cheese, and walnuts in a mixing bowl. In a small bowl, whisk together orange juice concentrate and olive oil. Pour mixture over salad and toss until fruit is coated.

Exchanges and Nutritional Analysis:
Exchanges: 1 dairy, 1 fruit, 1½ fat   Calcium (mg): 273
Calories: 200   % calories from carbohydrate: 34
% calories from protein: 18   % calories from fat: 48   Fiber (g): 2

Potato Salad

YIELD: 6 SERVINGS

1 pound small red potatoes,
  unpeeled
¼ cup finely chopped celery
¼ cup chopped red bell pepper
½ cup sliced green onion
¼ cup chopped cilantro

¾ cup nonfat plain yogurt
¾ cup nonfat dry milk powder
1 tablespoon Dijon mustard
¼ teaspoon black pepper
½ teaspoon salt
¼ teaspoon dried dill

Cook whole potatoes in boiling water until tender; drain and cool. Slice cooled potatoes into a mixing bowl. Add celery, bell pepper, onion, and cilantro to potatoes. In a separate bowl, mix yogurt and milk powder until smooth. Add mustard, pepper, salt, and dill. Pour yogurt dressing over potatoes and gently mix to combine.

Exchanges and Nutritional Analysis:
Exchanges: ½ dairy, 1 bread/grain   Calcium (mg): 181
Calories: 108   % calories from carbohydrate: 75
% calories from protein: 24   % calories from fat: 1   Fiber (g): 2

Sandwiches and Wraps

You'll find good nutrition and good taste packed between these slices of bread (or folded into the wrap). Each of these sandwiches can be the centerpiece of a satisfying meal.

Veggie and Cheese Sub Sandwich

YIELD: 4 SERVINGS

1 (8-ounce) loaf multigrain French
  bread
4 ounces provolone cheese, sliced
4 ounces reduced-fat cheddar
  cheese, sliced
1 cup finely shredded lettuce
½ cup very thinly sliced cucumber
¼ sweet onion, very thinly sliced

1 tomato, thinly sliced
1 tablespoon red wine vinegar
1 tablespoon olive oil
¼ teaspoon dried basil
¼ teaspoon dried oregano
¼ teaspoon salt
¼ teaspoon black pepper
¼ cup minced black olives

Cut French bread in half lengthwise; open loaf cut-side up. Scoop out and discard some of the inside bread on both sides of bread, leaving a shell. Arrange provolone slices along the length of one side of the loaf and arrange cheddar slices along the other side. Layer lettuce, cucumber, onion, and tomato down the center of the loaf. In a small bowl, whisk together vinegar, olive oil, basil, oregano, salt, and pepper. Add minced olives to dressing mixture and whisk. Pour mixture over sandwich. Fold halves of loaf together and cut into four pieces.

Exchanges and Nutritional Analysis:
Exchanges: 1½ dairy, 1 bread/grain, 1 vegetable, 2 fat
Calcium (mg): 499   Calories: 365   % calories from carbohydrate: 32
% calories from protein: 24   % calories from fat: 44   Fiber (g): 4

Grilled Turkey, Vegetable, and Cheese Sandwich

YIELD: 1 SERVING

2 (¾-ounce) slices reduced-fat cheddar cheese, divided
2 slices whole-wheat bread
1 roma tomato, sliced ¼ inch thick

1 ounce smoked deli turkey
¼ cup sliced roasted red peppers
1–2 tablespoons thinly sliced basil
1 teaspoon butter, softened

Lay one slice of cheese on one slice of bread. Top with tomato slices, turkey, peppers, and basil. Add remaining slice of cheese and place other slice of bread on top. Spread half the butter on top slice of bread. Grill sandwich, butter-side down, over medium heat until browned on the bottom. While cooking, spread remaining butter on top slice of bread. Turn sandwich; cook until browned and cheese is melted.

Exchanges and Nutritional Analysis:
Exchanges: 1½ dairy, 2 bread/grain, 1 meat/protein
Calcium (mg): 436   Calories: 338   % calories from carbohydrate: 35
% calories from protein: 27   % calories from fat: 38   Fiber (g): 5

Fattoush Pita

YIELD: 8 SERVINGS

1 cup finely chopped cucumber
½ cup finely chopped tomato
8 ounces crumbled feta cheese
¼ cup thinly sliced green onion
1½ cups thinly shredded romaine
   lettuce
1 cup thinly shredded spinach

¼ cup thinly shredded mint
1 tablespoon olive oil
2 tablespoons lemon juice
½ teaspoon salt
⅛ teaspoon black pepper
¼ teaspoon minced fresh garlic
4 (6-inch) whole-wheat pitas, halved

Combine cucumber, tomato, feta cheese, onion, lettuce, spinach, and mint in a mixing bowl. In a separate bowl, combine olive oil, lemon juice, salt, pepper, and garlic. Whisk well to combine dressing and pour over salad mixture. Spoon about ½ cup salad mixture into each pita half.

Exchanges and Nutritional Analysis:
Exchanges: ½ dairy, 1 bread/grain, 1 fat   Calcium (mg): 162
Calories: 180   % calories from carbohydrate: 42
% calories from protein: 16   % calories from fat: 41   Fiber (g): 3

Fajita Lettuce Wraps
YIELD: 6 SERVINGS

¼ teaspoon ground cumin
⅛ teaspoon chili powder
⅛ teaspoon dried oregano
2 cloves garlic, minced
¼ teaspoon salt
¼ teaspoon black pepper
⅛ teaspoon cayenne pepper
1 pound lean beef top sirloin
juice of 1 lime

¾ cup dry brown rice
1 (14-ounce) can Mexican-style
   tomatoes, juice reserved
1 (15-ounce) can black beans, rinsed
   and drained
⅓ cup chopped cilantro
1½ cups reduced-fat Mexican cheese
6 large Romaine lettuce leaves
salsa (optional)

Combine cumin, chili powder, oregano, garlic, salt, black pepper, and cayenne pepper in a small bowl. Rub spice mixture into beef and place in a glass dish or plastic storage bag. Squeeze lime juice over beef. Cover or seal and refrigerate for 2 hours. When ready to cook, preheat grill. Grill over medium-high heat until cooked to desired degree of doneness. Let stand a few minutes after cooking before slicing into thin strips.

Meanwhile, place rice in a saucepan. Drain juice from canned tomatoes into a measuring cup. Add enough water to equal 1½ cups liquid. Add liquid to rice. Bring to a boil. Reduce heat, cover, and simmer 20 to 30 minutes, or until tender. Chop drained tomatoes and gently mix into cooked rice along with black beans and cilantro.

To assemble each wrap, spoon about ¾ cup rice mixture down the center of a lettuce leaf. Add 2 ounces beef strips and ¼ cup cheese. Fold lettuce leaf around filling. Repeat with remaining ingredients. If desired, serve with salsa.

Exchanges and Nutritional Analysis:
Exchanges: 1 dairy, 1½ bread/grain, 1 vegetable, 2 meat/protein
Calcium (mg): 311   Calories: 351   % calories from carbohydrate: 39
% calories from protein: 36   % calories from fat: 26   Fiber (g): 6

Vegetable Dishes

Maybe you don't like cooked vegetables very much. But what if you added some delicious melted cheese? That's what every one of the recipes in this section does, giving the vegetable dishes a creamy taste that's hard to resist.

Tabbouleh Zucchini

YIELD: 6 SERVINGS

⅓ cup dry bulgur wheat
⅔ cup hot water
3 medium zucchini
¼ cup sliced green onions
2 tablespoons pine nuts
1 roma tomato, finely diced

2 tablespoons chopped fresh parsley
¼ teaspoon salt
¼ teaspoon black pepper
6 ounces feta cheese
¼ cup grated Parmesan cheese

Soak bulgur in hot water for 40 minutes or until plump. Drain and squeeze bulgur by hand to get rid of excess moisture. Measure out ½ cup and place in a mixing bowl. Meanwhile, cut each zucchini in half lengthwise and scoop out pulp, leaving a ¼-inch shell. Place shells in a baking dish. Add onions, pine nuts, tomato, parsley, salt, pepper, and feta cheese to bulgur in mixing bowl. Mix well. Spoon mixture into zucchini shells. Sprinkle Parmesan cheese on top. Bake at 350 degrees for 30 minutes or until zucchini are tender.

Exchanges and Nutritional Analysis:
Exchanges: ½ dairy, 1 vegetable, 1 fat   Calcium (mg): 205
Calories: 134   % calories from carbohydrate: 23
% calories from protein: 22   % calories from fat: 55   Fiber (g): 2

Tomato Pepper Penne

YIELD: 4 SERVINGS

1 (14½-ounce) can Italian-style
   tomatoes, undrained
1 (7-ounce) jar roasted red peppers,
   drained
3 cloves garlic
1 teaspoon olive oil
¼ teaspoon paprika
1 teaspoon dried basil

7 ounces dry whole-wheat penne
   pasta (½ package)
½ cup fat-free half-and-half
1 cup reduced-fat Monterey Jack
   cheese
1 (2¼-ounce) can sliced black
   olives, drained
¼ cup grated Parmesan cheese

Process tomatoes and peppers in a blender until pureed. In a skillet, sauté garlic in oil until softened. Add tomato mixture, paprika, and basil. Bring mixture to a boil. Reduce heat to a simmer and cook 10 to 15 minutes to reduce sauce. Meanwhile, cook pasta in boiling water until al dente; drain. Stir half-and-half into reduced sauce and remove from heat. Combine sauce, pasta, Monterey Jack cheese, and olives in a mixing bowl. Toss until cheese melts. Transfer to a serving bowl. Sprinkle with Parmesan cheese.

Exchanges and Nutritional Analysis:
Exchanges: 1½ dairy, 2 bread/grain, 1 vegetable   Calcium (mg): 451
Calories: 368   % calories from carbohydrate: 55
% calories from protein: 21   % calories from fat: 24   Fiber (g): 6

Stuffed Tomatoes
YIELD: 4 SERVINGS

4 large tomatoes
1 cup dry herb stuffing
1½ cups low-fat ricotta cheese

2 tablespoons chopped parsley
½ cup Parmesan cheese, divided

Cut out stem of each tomato; scoop out and discard seeds and pulp; set tomato shells aside. In a mixing bowl, combine stuffing, ricotta cheese, parsley, and 6 tablespoons Parmesan cheese. Spoon mixture loosely into tomato shells. Place in a baking dish and sprinkle remaining 2 tablespoons Parmesan cheese on top. Bake at 350 degrees for 30 minutes or until bubbly and starting to brown.

Exchanges and Nutritional Analysis:
Exchanges: 1 dairy, ½ bread/grain, 1 vegetable, 1 fat
Calcium (mg): 313   Calories: 231   % calories from carbohydrate: 43
% calories from protein: 26   % calories from fat: 31   Fiber (g): 3

Sweet Potatoes on the Half Shell
YIELD: 4 SERVINGS

2 (12-ounce) sweet potatoes
¼ cup dry milk powder
2 tablespoons milk

½ cup low-fat cottage cheese
⅛ teaspoon cinnamon

Bake or microwave sweet potatoes until soft, then cut in half lengthwise. Scoop out potato pulp into a mixing bowl, leaving a ¼-inch-thick shell; set shells aside. Combine dry milk powder and milk and stir until dissolved. Add milk mixture, cottage cheese, and brown sugar to potato pulp. Beat with a hand mixer until smooth. Spoon mixture into potato shells. For added effect, add the last third of mixture through a piping bag fitted with a decorating tip. Lightly dust cinnamon on top. Bake at 350 degrees for 20 to 30 minutes or until hot.

Exchanges and Nutritional Analysis:
Exchanges: ½ dairy, 2½ bread/grain   Calcium (mg): 131
Calories: 215   % calories from carbohydrate: 84
% calories from protein: 15   % calories from fat: 1   Fiber (g): 5

Portabella Mushroom Burgers with Caramelized Balsamic Onions
YIELD: 4 SERVINGS

Burgers:
1 tablespoon olive oil
½ teaspoon salt
½ teaspoon black pepper
1 tablespoon white wine
1 teaspoon Worcestershire sauce
4 (4-inch) portabella mushroom caps, stems removed

4 (1-ounce) slices reduced-fat Swiss cheese
4 whole-wheat sandwich buns
4 lettuce leaves
4 tomato slices

Caramelized Balsamic Onions:
½ teaspoon olive oil
1½ cups sliced onions

1 tablespoon balsamic vinegar
¼ teaspoon salt

Combine olive oil, salt, pepper, wine, and Worcestershire sauce. Set aside while preparing remainder of recipe to give flavors time to meld. To prepare onions, heat oil in a small saucepan over medium heat. Add onions and sauté until softened. Cook, stirring occasionally, for 10 to 15 minutes. Stir in vinegar and salt and cook until vinegar evaporates. When ready to cook the mushrooms, preheat grill. Brush top of each mushroom cap and the border around the bottom of cap with olive oil mixture. Place caps on grill over medium heat, top side up. Cook 3 minutes or until mushrooms start to brown around the edges. Turn and cook another 3 minutes or until softened and browned and juices are accumulating where the stem was. Turn caps again so that tops are upward. Place a slice of cheese on each cap and cook until cheese melts. Toast buns briefly on grill. Place a cap on each bun and top with lettuce and tomato slice. Serve topped with Caramelized Balsamic Onions.

Exchanges and Nutritional Analysis:
Exchanges: 1 dairy, 1½ bread/grain, 1 vegetable, 1 fat
Calcium (mg): 333   Calories: 273   % calories from carbohydrate: 46
% calories from protein: 20   % calories from fat: 33   Fiber (g): 5

Eggplant Lasagna
YIELD: 8 SERVINGS

¼ cup chopped onion
1 clove garlic, minced
1 teaspoon olive oil
1 (14½-ounce) can Italian-style diced tomatoes, undrained
2 pounds fresh roma tomatoes, peeled, seeded, and coarsely chopped
1 tablespoon minced basil
½ teaspoon salt

1 large (1 to 1¼-pound) eggplant
8 ounces portabella mushroom caps
1 egg white
1 (15-ounce) container light ricotta cheese
1 cup shredded reduced-fat mozzarella cheese
½ cup grated Parmesan cheese, divided

Sauté onion and garlic in olive oil until softened. Puree undrained canned tomatoes with a hand blender or in a food processor. Add pureed tomatoes and chopped fresh tomatoes to sautéed onion. Season with basil and salt. Simmer, uncovered, over medium heat for 15 to 20 minutes.

Meanwhile, peel eggplant and cut into ¼-inch-thick lengthwise slices. Slice mushroom caps ¼-inch-thick. In a mixing bowl, lightly beat egg white. Add ricotta cheese, mozzarella cheese, and ¼ cup Parmesan cheese and mix well.

To assemble lasagna, spread ½ cup of tomato sauce in the bottom of a 9 × 13–inch glass baking dish. Top with a single layer of eggplant slices, then a single layer of mushroom slices. Spoon 1 cup tomato sauce on top. Spread half of the cheese mixture over the sauce. Add another layer of eggplant, then mushrooms, using remaining mushrooms, 1 cup sauce, and remainder of cheese mixture. Top with a final layer of eggplant. Spoon remaining sauce over eggplant and sprinkle with remaining ¼ cup Parmesan cheese. Bake at 350 degrees for 50 minutes. Remove from oven and let stand 10 minutes before cutting.

Exchanges and Nutritional Analysis:
Exchanges: 1 dairy, 2 vegetable, 1 fat   Calcium (mg): 284
Calories: 182   % calories from carbohydrate: 39
% calories from protein: 27   % calories from fat: 34   Fiber (g): 3

Creamy Mashed Potatoes

YIELD: 6 SERVINGS

2½ pounds russet potatoes, peeled
and cut into large chunks
4 cloves garlic, peeled
1 cup nonfat dry milk powder

½ teaspoon salt
¾ cup fat-free half-and-half, warmed
¾ cup shredded fontina cheese

Cook potatoes and whole garlic cloves in boiling water in a large saucepan until tender. Drain and return to pan. Dissolve milk powder and salt in half-and-half and add to potatoes and garlic. Use an electric beater to blend mixture until smooth. Stir in cheese until melted.

Exchanges and Nutritional Analysis:
Exchanges: 1 dairy, 2 bread/grain   Calcium (mg): 283
Calories: 244   % calories from carbohydrate: 64
% calories from protein: 21   % calories from fat: 14   Fiber (g): 4

Fruit Dishes

In our studies at the University of Tennessee, people on the Calcium Key Weight-Loss Plan sometimes find that one of their biggest challenges is getting all their daily fruit exchanges. Most of us just aren't accustomed to eating a lot of fruit. These recipes make it easier.

Fresh Fruit Kebobs with Citrus Poppy-Seed Dressing

YIELD: 4 SERVINGS

4 cups fruit pieces of your choice
½ cup nonfat plain yogurt
½ cup nonfat dry milk powder
½ teaspoon lemon juice

½ teaspoon lime juice
½ teaspoon lemon zest
1 tablespoon Splenda Granular
¼ teaspoon poppy seeds

Thread fruit pieces onto 8 skewers. In a small mixing bowl, combine yogurt and milk powder and mix until smooth. Add lemon juice, lime juice, lemon zest, Splenda and poppy seeds. Serve yogurt dressing on the side as a dipping sauce for the kebobs.

Exchanges and Nutritional Analysis:
Exchanges: ½ dairy, 1 fruit   Calcium (mg): 186
Calories: 119   % calories from carbohydrate: 76
% calories from protein: 18   % calories from fat: 6   Fiber (g): 3

Frozen Fruit Cups

YIELD: 6 SERVINGS

1 cup nonfat plain yogurt
1¼ cups nonfat dry milk powder
4 ounces Neufchâtel cheese, softened
1 tablespoon Splenda Granular
1 (8-ounce) can crushed pineapple in juice, drained

2 cups sliced strawberries
1 cup blueberries
1 peach, peeled and sliced
1 cup seedless grapes
6 lettuce leaves for garnish

Combine yogurt and milk powder in a mixing bowl and stir until smooth. Blend in Neufchâtel cheese and Splenda until smooth. Stir in drained pineapple. Add strawberries, blueberries, peach slices, and grapes and mix. Spoon mixture into 6 large (1-cup) muffin cups. Freeze 4 hours or until firm. When ready to serve, dip bottom of muffin tin in warm water briefly to loosen salad. Unmold onto individual lettuce-lined plates.

Exchanges and Nutritional Analysis:
Exchanges: 1 dairy, 1½ fruit, ½ fat   Calcium (mg): 281
Calories: 197   % calories from carbohydrate: 59
% calories from protein: 20   % calories from fat: 21   Fiber (g): 3

Desserts

Sautéed Apple Crepes

YIELD: 6 SERVINGS

Crepes:
½ cup all-purpose flour
¼ cup whole-wheat flour
½ tablespoon sugar
¼ teaspoon baking powder
¼ teaspoon salt

¼ cup nonfat dry milk powder
1 cup milk
1 egg
1 teaspoon butter, melted
¼ teaspoon vanilla extract

Apples:
2 cups peeled and chopped apples
1 teaspoon butter

2 teaspoons sugar
¼ teaspoon cinnamon

Topping:
¾ cup nonfat plain yogurt

2 tablespoons sugar
¼ teaspoon cinnamon

To make crepe, combine flours, sugar, baking powder, and salt in a mixing bowl. Dissolve milk powder in milk. Beat milk mixture, egg, butter, and vanilla extract into dry ingredients until smooth. Cook crepes over medium heat in a nonstick skillet by pouring ¼ cup of batter into hot skillet. Tilt skillet to spread batter and cook until lightly browned on bottom. Carefully turn crepe and cook until lightly browned on other side. Stack crepes as they finish cooking, separating them with wax paper; keep warm.

To make apples, sauté chopped apples in butter until they start to soften. Combine sugar and cinnamon and sprinkle over apples. Toss and sauté until cinnamon mixture evenly coats apples and apples are just tender; do not overcook.

For topping, mix together yogurt, sugar, and cinnamon. To assemble, spoon ¼ cup hot apple filling into center of each warm crepe. Fold in sides of crepes around filling and place on individual serving plates. Spoon 2 tablespoons topping over each crepe.

Exchanges and Nutritional Analysis:
Exchanges: ½ dairy, 1 bread/grain, ½ fruit
Calcium (mg): 169   Calories: 168   % calories from carbohydrate: 70
% calories from protein: 16   % calories from fat: 14   Fiber (g): 2

Fruit Pizza

YIELD: 12 SERVINGS

1 (14-ounce) can fat-free sweetened condensed milk
½ cup plus 2 tablespoons non-fat plain yogurt, divided
¼ cup fresh lemon juice
½ teaspoon vanilla extract
6 tablespoons butter, softened

¼ cup brown sugar
¾ cup all-purpose flour
½ cup quick-cooking oats
4 cups assorted fruit such as sliced strawberries, kiwi, blueberries, and canned mandarin orange slices

To make filling, combine milk, ½ cup yogurt, lemon juice, and vanilla extract in a small mixing bowl. Mix well and chill until thickened. In a large mixing bowl, cream butter, 2 tablespoons yogurt, and brown sugar until fluffy. Add flour and oats. Blend well. Press dough into an 11-inch circle on a lightly greased pizza pan or baking sheet. Bake at 350 degrees for 15 minutes or until golden brown. Cool and carefully transfer to a flat serving platter. When ready to serve, spoon chilled filling evenly over cooled crust. Arrange fruit in a decorative pattern on filling and cut into wedges.

Exchanges and Nutritional Analysis:
Exchanges: ½ dairy, 1 bread/grain, 1½ fruit, ½ fat
Calcium (mg): 132   Calories: 238   % calories from carbohydrate: 68
% calories from protein: 9   % calories from fat: 23   Fiber (g): 2

6

Burn More Fat with Easy Exercise

YOU DON'T NEED TO exercise to lose weight on the Calcium Key Weight-Loss Plan. Dairy foods change how your fat cells work, whether you exercise or not. Eating 3 to 4 servings of dairy a day will trigger your fat cells to make less fat, burn more fat, and store less fat.

But even though you don't need to exercise to lose weight on the plan, I strongly encourage you to do so. Every time you move your muscles, you burn more calories, which means exercise can help you lose weight. It can also strengthen your heart, muscles, and bones, boost your energy, and brighten your mood. And studies show that exercise may be a key factor in long-term weight-loss success.

Let's look at the evidence that exercising regularly is a smart idea if you want to be thinner today, and for the rest of your life.

Exercise: A Proven Formula for Burning Fat

Remember The Calorie Equation from chapter 2?

- If you take in more calories than you burn, you will gain weight.
- If you burn more calories than you take in, you will lose weight.

Exercise burns calories. If you exercise regularly, it's likely you'll burn more calories than you take in and shed some additional pounds. Regular exercise can help you keep the pounds off, too. Let's look at the research.

Exercise Helps You Keep the Weight Off

Researchers at the University of Kentucky analyzed six studies on long-term weight-loss maintenance (4 to 5 years after weight loss) and exercise.

Writing about their findings in the *American Journal of Clinical Nutrition,* they note that people who exercise more have significantly greater weight-loss maintenance than people who exercise less. On average, 53% of those who do more exercise keep off their weight, compared to 27% of those who do less. Regular exercise almost doubles the success rate of long-term weight-loss maintenance!

Exercise Helps Dieters Stay Happy

Exercise may also help you stay happier while you're cutting calories. In a study published in the *Journal of Psychosomatic Research,* scientists measured psychological general well-being in four groups of overweight women. The four groups were either (1) not dieting or exercising, (2) dieting, (3) exercising, or (4) dieting and exercising.

The women who were dieting and exercising had the greatest sense of well-being. They felt freer from worries and concerns about their health, more cheerful than depressed, more relaxed than tense, even more satisfied with life.

Exercise may also improve your ability to stick with a diet. In a study of 264 dieters conducted by scientists at Stanford University School of Medicine and published in *Obesity Research,* those who exercised found it easier not to overeat than those who didn't exercise. It's possible that the exercisers felt less hungry during the day.

Choosing the Exercise That's Right for You

Let's say you've decided to exercise. Now you've got two more choices: the type of exercise you're going to do and the amount of time you're going to do it. Scientists have compiled a lot of evidence about the best type and amount of exercise for dieters.

Regular Exercise Is Key

To get the most up-to-date, accurate, and science-based advice about exercise and weight loss, I talked with a fellow faculty member at the University of Tennessee, Dr. Dixie Thompson, Ph.D., associate professor and the director of the Center for Physical Activity and Health in the Department of Health and Exercise Science. Thompson is a Fellow of the American College of Sports Medicine, the top professional organization in exercise science.

"There is no magic exercise for weight loss," says Thompson. Almost any calorie-burning exercise that you are willing to do regularly will help you lose weight. So how do you make sure you exercise regularly?

Find a support system, she advises. Your support system can be just one person you can count on to exercise with you or a group of friends who exercise together. Agree on a specific time and place to exercise together—for example, Monday, Wednesday, and Friday evenings at six for a 30-minute walk in the local park. "The scientific data are very strong that if you have one or more supportive people helping you stick with an exercise program, you're much more likely to become a regular exerciser," says Thompson.

Another key to regular exercise: make sure the significant people in your life understand that exercise time is *your* time. For example, says Thompson, "Before you exercise, tell your kids, 'The next 45 minutes is Mom's time. If you need anything, talk to Dad.'"

Another strategy that sometimes helps people exercise regularly is a financial commitment. "Join a gym or health club and work out there," says Thompson. Or invest in a good pair of walking shoes or home exercise equipment. "Because you've made a literal investment in exercise, you may be more likely to stick with it."

But maybe all these tips about turning yourself into a regular exerciser don't sound like they'll work because you've tried to exercise regularly and never found it much fun. "Give regular exercise one more *extended* try," says Dr. Thompson.

"Again and again, I've seen people discover that exercise is enjoyable, but it almost always takes a little time," she says. Maybe you won't enjoy exercising for a week or two. Maybe not even for the first month. But after 6 weeks to 2 months, you'll begin to experience benefits that will motivate you to keep going. You'll feel healthier. You'll look better. And because you've adopted a new, healthy habit, you're likely to feel better about yourself.

"If you can get through those first couple of weeks and adapt to a routine of regular exercise," says Thompson, "it's likely you'll keep exercising for the rest of your life."

Moderate-Intensity Exercise—Just Right

How hard should you exercise? Should you push yourself to the point where you don't think you can keep going anymore? Or should you take it easy, barely breaking a sweat?

Exercise physiologists say the best way to exercise for weight loss is at a moderate-intensity level. In scientific terms, this means exercising at 55 to 69% of your maximum heart rate. However, without special tests to determine your maximum heart rate and devices to monitor your rate during exercise, how do you know for certain whether you're in the 55–69% range? Fortunately, says Thompson, there's an easy way to figure out whether your exercise is at a moderate-intensity level.

"Your own perception of how intensely you're exercising is an accurate way to determine if you're at a low-, moderate-, or high-intensity level," she says.

Ask yourself the following questions about the exercise you're doing. If it's moderate intensity, you'll answer yes to questions 1, 2, and 3, and no to questions 4 and 5.

1. Am I exercising intensely enough to sweat?
2. Am I exercising intensely enough to breathe hard?
3. If I exercise for 30 to 45 minutes, do I feel a little tired immediately afterward and refreshed about an hour later?
4. Do I feel so breathless that I can't speak? (If yes, the exercise is high rather than moderate intensity.)
5. Do I feel exhausted immediately afterward and not refreshed later? (If yes, the exercise is high rather than moderate intensity.)

It's not that high-intensity exercise is bad for you, says Thompson. In fact, compared to moderate intensity, it burns more calories in the same amount of time. But moderate-intensity exercise is what you are most likely to do on a regular basis, particularly if you're trying to make the switch from being a sedentary person to a regular exerciser. For most people, moderate-intensity exercise is the most realistic type of exercise to help achieve weight loss, she says.

There are many types of exercise you can do at a moderate pace. They include brisk walking, jogging, bicycling, swimming, racquetball, tennis, and exercises using a machine, such as a treadmill, stairclimber, or rowing machine.

150 Minutes per Week

Studies show that for long-term maintenance of weight loss, you need to exercise at least 150 minutes a week. That might sound like a lot, but it's not—it's just 30 minutes 5 days a week.

However, it's also good to keep in mind that 150 minutes a week of exercise is the *minimum* amount of exercise you need to maintain weight loss. Studies also show that 300 minutes a week (60 minutes 5 days a week) is more likely to keep weight off for a lifetime.

Moderate-intensity walking, or brisk walking, may be the best exercise for helping you lose weight, says Thompson. You don't need any special equipment, just a good pair of walking shoes. You don't need to learn special skills, as you would if you decided to take up tennis as your regular exercise. You can walk just about anytime, anywhere. And walking is easy on your joints (unlike jogging, for example), which is an important factor to consider if you're carrying around extra pounds.

Thompson describes this easy-to-follow walking program: Begin each exercise session with a warm-up walk at a comfortable pace. For the first week, walk 15 minutes—10 minutes at your comfortable pace, then 5 minutes a bit more briskly. The second week, increase your total amount of walking time by 10%. The third week, keep your total walking time the same, but increase the time you walk briskly by 10%. Continue that pattern of 10% increases week by week. Based on these guidelines, a 20-week walking program would look something like this:

Week 1:   15 minutes total/5 minutes brisk
Week 2:   17 minutes total/5 minutes brisk
Week 3:   17 minutes total/6 minutes brisk
Week 4:   19 minutes total/6 minutes brisk
Week 5:   19 minutes total/7 minutes brisk
Week 6:   21 minutes total/7 minutes brisk
Week 7:   21 minutes total/9 minutes brisk
Week 8:   23 minutes total/9 minutes brisk
Week 9:   23 minutes total/10 minutes brisk
Week 10:   25 minutes total/10 minutes brisk
Week 11:   25 minutes total/11 minutes brisk
Week 12:   27 minutes total/11 minutes brisk
Week 13:   27 minutes total/12 minutes brisk
Week 14:   30 minutes total/12 minutes brisk
Week 15:   30 minutes total/15 minutes brisk
Week 16:   30 minutes total/17 minutes brisk
Week 17:   30 minutes total/20 minutes brisk
Week 18:   30 minutes total/22 minutes brisk
Week 19:   30 minutes total/25 minutes brisk
Week 20:   30 minutes total/30 minutes brisk

Of course, you'll want to adjust the program to your own abilities and inclinations. Some people will find walking briskly for 5 minutes the first week a challenge. Others might start walking briskly for the entire 15 minutes. If you can, it's always best to meet with a trained fitness expert to help you individualize your exercise program.

If you have heart disease, diabetes, or another serious medical condition, talk with your doctor before beginning an exercise program. If you begin walking and notice any unusual symptoms, such as chest pain or difficulty breathing, consult your physician immediately; these are signs of heart disease.

Intermittent Exercise: Fitness 10 Minutes at a Time

Maybe you think an exercise session has to last a long time for it to do you any good. The latest research in exercise science shows that shorter or intermittent bouts of exercise are just as effective as longer bouts.

That's right—exercising for 10 minutes three times a day can help you lose weight just as effectively as exercising for 30 minutes all at once. If you find it hard to fit a longer bout of exercise into a busy schedule, this could make all the difference in whether you exercise regularly. Does this shorter-is-okay idea sound too good to be true? Take a look at some of the scientific evidence.

In a study reported in the *Journal of the American Medical Association,* researchers from Brown University School of Medicine put 115 overweight women on an 18-month exercise program, separating them into three groups. One group did long-bout exercise: 40 minutes of walking in one session 5 days a week. A second group did short-bout exercise: 40 minutes of walking divided into four 10-minute sessions 5 days a week. A third group also did short-bout exercise but used a motorized treadmill.

After 18 months, the average weight loss in the short-bout treadmill group was 16 pounds, in the long-bout walking group 13 pounds, and in the short-bout walking group 8 pounds. This difference between the groups wasn't based on the type of exercise; it turned out that the women who had exercise equipment at home exercised more regularly. Whether the women exercised in short bouts or long bouts didn't make any difference in weight loss: both short-bout and long-bout exercise was effective *if* the women exercised. The researchers did find, however, that the more the women exercised, the more weight they lost, with those exercising over 200 minutes a week losing far more weight than those who exercised less than 150 minutes a week.

In another study conducted by Finnish scientists and reported in the *Scandinavian Journal of Medicine and Science in Sports,* 134 postmenopausal women exercised 5 days a week at moderate intensity. One group exercised in a single session; another group exercised in two sessions a day. After 15 weeks, the levels of weight loss and fat loss in the two groups were virtually the same. And fitness levels—what the scientists called "aerobic power"—also improved at the same rate.

"Exercise improved the maximal aerobic power and body composition [weight and fat] equally when walking was performed in one or two daily bouts," write the researchers. I want you to feel confident that you can get all of the weight-reducing benefits of exercise even if you choose frequent, short bouts rather than one long bout.

And, along with shorter bouts of exercise, there's another easy way to burn calories and lose weight. Scientists call it "lifestyle activity," or simply the activities of daily living, like walking the dog.

The Activities of Daily Living: A Great Way to Burn Calories

Why circle the mall looking for the "best" (the closest) parking spot? Really, when we're talking about the best way to take off and keep off pounds, the best parking spot in the lot is the one that's farthest away from the mall entrance. The little bit of extra walking you'll add to your day by parking farther away from the entrance is going to burn a few more calories.

You can also burn a few more calories by taking the stairs rather than the escalator . . . by pushing a lawnmower rather than riding one . . . by raking rather than blowing leaves . . . by getting out of the car at the fast-food restaurant rather than using the drive-through. Little by little, all of these calorie-burning daily activities add up, leading to better weight control.

In a study reported in the *Journal of the American Medical Association*, researchers from the Johns Hopkins University School of Medicine looked at two groups of women who weighed an average of 196 pounds. Both groups were put on a low-calorie diet. But the two groups did very different types of physical activity.

One group attended step aerobic classes three times a week, building up to 45 minutes of exercise per session by the eighth week of the study. Researchers instructed the other group to increase their activities of daily living: to walk short distances rather than drive, for example, and to take the stairs rather than the elevator or escalator.

After 4 months, the aerobic group had lost an average of 19 pounds and the lifestyle group had lost an average of 17. So, there was almost no difference in weight loss between the women who exercised regularly and the women who had increased their daily activities.

There are many other activities of daily living besides walking. A short list includes gardening, golfing without a cart, shoveling snow, mowing with a push mower, sweeping and other types of housework, pushing a baby stroller, and raking leaves.

And remember that your decision to increase activities of daily living doesn't have to be all or nothing. For example, maybe you work on the 10th floor of an office building and would find it too difficult to walk up all 10 flights on your way to work. Instead, walk up one flight and take the elevator the rest of the way. After a few weeks, walk up two flights before taking the elevator. You could also consider walking down the stairs on your way out of the office.

Try a Pedometer

One approach I'd like to recommend to help you increase your activities of daily living is to wear a step counter, or pedometer. This small device is worn on your hip and measures the number of steps you take. Thompson has done extensive research on pedometers and health. In one of her studies, postmenopausal women who were given pedometers and asked to increase their daily steps by 4000 a day were able to lower their blood pressure by an average of 11 points—a drop as large as that achieved by pressure-lowering drugs.

Thompson says that not all pedometers are created equal. You need to purchase a device that you're sure is accurate. Buy one with a money-back guarantee, put it on, and take about 20 counted steps in an area where you typically walk, like a carpeted area at work or in your backyard at home. See if the pedometer counted the same number of steps as you did. If not, return it, buy another model, and repeat the test.

Once you've found an accurate pedometer, wear it for a week when you're not trying to increase your lifestyle activities. At the end of each day, record your total number of steps. After the week is over, compute your daily average. This gives you a baseline amount for the number of steps you typically take in a day.

Then start to gradually increase the amount of steps you walk a day. For example, park a block away from work rather than in the company parking lot. Take the stairs rather than the elevator to your office (or at least take the stairs up a flight or two). How many more steps per day are you trying to achieve?

There are 2000 to 2500 steps in a mile. Try to increase your daily average by at least that much. If you increase by 4000 to 5000 steps, you'll walk an extra 2 miles a day—exactly the distance it would take you for 30 minutes walking at a brisk pace. By increasing your activities of daily living, you can increase the amount of walking you do each day to the same level that experts say is the minimum for maintaining weight loss.

Resistance Training: Tone Your Body

Resistance training—working out with weights—is a smart part of any weight-loss program. But not because it helps you lose weight. Yes, it can increase and tone muscle, perhaps triggering a small boost in metabolism, the rate at which your body burns calories. Yes, it builds your strength, boosting your physical capacities and mental confidence. And, yes, as you age, you'll have stronger bones and therefore be less likely to suffer a disabling injury that can rob you of independence.

But studies show that resistance training won't help you lose weight. Compared to aerobic exercises like walking, resistance training burns relatively few calories. Resistance training isn't a necessary part of the Calcium Key Weight-Loss Plan. But we certainly encourage anyone interested in this form of healthful exercise to investigate it further.

There are many types of resistance training: working out on a weight machine like a Nautilus; using free weights, like dumbbells and barbells; or just doing calisthenics, like a pushup, where the weight of the body is the resistance. There are also many different routines for resistance training available, such as those popularized in *Strong Women* books by Miriam E. Nelson, Ph.D., professor at Tufts University.

The American College of Sports Medicine recommends that a person beginning resistance training—a healthy adult who isn't currently exercising regularly—do at least one set (10 to 12 repetitions) of 8 to 10 resistance exercises twice a week. That's a good, scientifically proven guideline for you to follow.

Regular exercise burns calories. And that can only help boost the remarkable calorie-burning power of the Calcium Key Weight-Loss Plan.

PART III

OTHER HEALTH BENEFITS OF THE CALCIUM KEY WEIGHT-LOSS PLAN

7

Gaining Health While Losing Weight

How Calcium Can Protect You from Osteoporosis, High Blood Pressure, Colon Cancer, PMS, Polycystic Ovarian Syndrome, and Other Health Problems

YOU'RE READING THIS BOOK because you want to lose weight. And, if you follow the Calcium Key Weight-Loss Plan, you will lose weight. But the dairy foods and their rich cargo of calcium will affect a wide array of other cells in your body in addition to fat cells. Here's why.

Calcium molecules bind to many cell proteins—the worker bees of the cellular hive—helping form their structures so that they can do a variety of the body's basic tasks, like cell division, nerve transmission, and hormone secretion. And what happens to your body's cells also happens to your body's systems. A high calcium-diet

- Affects the *circulatory system*, relaxing the muscle walls of arteries, lowering blood pressure, and helping prevent stroke and maybe heart disease
- Affects your hormone-manufacturing *endocrine system*, helping to regulate hormones and ease conditions like premenstrual syndrome, polycystic ovarian syndrome, and postpartum depression
- Affects how cells divide in many systems of your body, including your *digestive system*, thereby helping prevent the uncontrolled cell division that leads to colon cancer
- Affects your *skeletal system*, where calcium's role isn't as an assistant in manufacturing cellular proteins but is one of the key building materials of bone

The Calcium Key Weight-Loss Plan won't only help you lose weight day by day; it will also help you gain health. And that's what this chapter is all about.

Strong Bones Need Calcium

There's one part of your body that you don't want to get thinner—your bones. But that's exactly what happens in osteoporosis, when thick, sturdy bones become thin and fragile. The disease isn't an inevitable part of aging, as many believe. But it's very common. Ten million Americans have osteoporosis, 80% of whom are women. Another 34 million have osteopenia—low bone mass that is a possible prelude to osteoporosis. (Unlike osteoporosis, you can reverse osteopenia.) The result of all that bone thinning is that one of every two American women will suffer an osteoporosis-related bone fracture, most likely of a wrist, vertebra, or hip. Twenty-four percent of those over 50 who have hip fractures will die within the year, often of pneumonia or other complications. That's as many women as are killed each year by breast cancer. As for American men, 80,000 suffer a hip fracture every year, with one-third dying within the following 12 months.

There is scientific agreement on the best prevention for osteoporosis: calcium. That agreement is summarized in the consensus statement of the National Institutes of Health Conference on Osteoporosis Prevention, Diagnosis, and Therapy: "Adequate calcium and vitamin D intake [which helps the body absorb calcium] are crucial to develop optimal peak bone mass and to preserve bone mass throughout life."

For optimal bone health, every woman under age 51 needs 1000 milligrams (mg) of calcium a day, the amount in about $2^1/_2$ servings of dairy foods. But few get it. There isn't a single population of women in North America that, on average, meets the requirements for a level of calcium intake that can prevent osteoporosis. In fact, national nutrition surveys show that most people—women and men—consume less than half the calcium necessary to build and maintain healthy bones. And it's a low intake of dairy foods, the major dietary source of calcium, that's largely responsible for North Americans' low calcium intake.

Among kids and teens, the numbers are particularly dismal. Among 9- to 17-year-olds, only about 10% of girls and 25% of boys get the recommended 1300 mg of calcium a day. That low level of intake is very likely setting the stage for osteoporosis.

In a study in the January 2003 issue of the *American Journal of Clinical*

Nutrition, scientists at Children's Medical Center in Cincinnati looked at 3251 women, finding out their current bone mineral content (the best measure of a bone's strength) and their lifetime milk consumption. They discovered that women 29 to 49 years old who got less than 1 serving of dairy a day during childhood had a significantly lower bone mineral content than women who got more than 1 serving. When the scientists looked at milk drinking during adolescence, they once again found that women who got 1 serving or less had a lower level of bone minerals.

Low mineral content translates into thinner, weaker, more fracture-prone bones. Among women over 50 in the study, those who had a low milk intake during childhood were twice as likely to have a hip fracture.

Menopause and Your Bones

The onset of menopause, accompanied by falling estrogen levels, is a critical time for bones. Estrogen acts as a kind of warden that keeps calcium locked in the skeleton. When that hormone ebbs, the mineral escapes—for 5 years after the onset of menopause, bones rapidly lose density. That's why at menopause the daily calcium goal rises from 1000 to 1200 mg. And while calcium alone will not prevent bone loss after menopause, it plays a big role. An analysis of 15 studies of calcium intake and osteoporosis in postmenopausal women shows that higher calcium intake reduces bone loss in the spine by 36% and in the hip by 9%, reducing the risk of spinal fractures by 23% and of hip and other fractures by 14%. In a recent study of postmenopausal women published in the *Journal of the American Dietetic Association,* those who ate a snack of yogurt three times a day had a significantly lower rate of bone breakdown than those who ate a jellied candy three times a day.

Low Calcium, High Blood Pressure

Remember calcitriol, the hormone you read about in chapter 1? A low-calcium diet triggers increased levels of calcitriol, which allows more calcium into fat cells, and activates fat production and storage.

Calcitriol also affects the amount of calcium in the smooth muscle cells of your arteries—the cells that contract or relax the artery, controlling its width. When a low-calcium diet causes calcium to enter those cells, the calcium makes them contract, narrowing the artery. When an artery narrows, blood pressure increases—just as narrowing a garden hose while watering would increase the water pressure. Higher blood pressure, or hypertension, is bad news for your health.

The fast, turbulent flow of blood under pressure slowly but surely damages the walls of arteries, making the formation of fatty sores called *plaques* more likely. Those plaques can form blood clots. And if a clot blocks an artery, you're in trouble. A clot that blocks the flow of blood to the heart causes a heart attack. A clot that blocks the flow of blood to the brain causes a stroke. That's why artery-damaging, clot-causing hypertension is a leading risk factor for both heart disease and stroke, the #1 and #3 killers of North Americans. Fifty million Americans—one out of every four adults—have high blood pressure. Among those over 65, one out of every two people is hypertensive. If you're one of those millions, it's quite likely that the Calcium Key Weight-Loss Plan can help bring your pressure down.

Improving Your Numbers

Blood pressure is measured with two numbers: systolic and diastolic. Systolic shows the pressure in your blood vessels when the heart is pumping blood; diastolic, when the heart is relaxed. According to the most recent guidelines from the National Health, Lung, and Blood Institute of the National Institutes of Health,

- Normal blood pressure is less than 120 systolic and 80 diastolic, or less than 120/80
- Prehypertension—a situation where you don't have high blood pressure but are at increased risk for heart disease—is 120/80 to 139/89
- Hypertension is 140/90 or above

In those with hypertension, lowering systolic pressure by just 10 points can reduce the risk of stroke by 44% and the risk of a heart attack by 21%. A number of studies show that adding dairy to the diet can lower blood pressure. In a study in *Nutrition Reports International,* researchers substituted a quart of calcium-fortified skim milk for other beverages; among 27 people with high blood pressure, systolic pressure fell 9 points and diastolic 3. In a study involving 7 hypertensive men reported in the *Journal of the American Medical Association,* those who got 1500 mg a day of calcium from dairy products had a systolic pressure 9 points lower than men getting 400 mg of calcium. And in one of my own earlier studies on people with hypertension published in the *Journal of Hypertension* and in the *American Journal of Hypertension,* I found that 2 servings of yogurt containing 600 mg of calcium were substantially more effective in lowering blood pressure than 600 mg of calcium from supplements.

The DASH Study

The best evidence for the pressure-lowering power of dairy foods is the DASH Study: Dietary Approaches to Stop Hypertension. In this scientific investigation conducted at research centers across the United States in the late 1990s, people ate one of three diets for 8 weeks: (1) a control diet similar to the typical American diet; (2) a fruits and vegetables diet, with 8 servings of those foods a day; or (3) a combination diet with 8 servings of fruits and vegetables *and* low-fat dairy foods. The dairy foods included daily servings of 12 ounces of low-fat or fat-free milk, 3 ounces of yogurt, and 1.4 ounces of cheese—3 servings of dairy a day, the same as in the Calcium Key Weight-Loss Plan. The calories were the same for all three diets, as was the level of salt or sodium.

For the hypertensives in the study, the combination diet emphasizing fruits, vegetables, and low-fat dairy products reduced systolic blood pressure by an average of 11.4 points—the same reduction typically achieved by taking medication for high blood pressure. In contrast, the fruits and vegetables diet reduced systolic blood pressure by an average of only 2.8 points. The authors of the study say, "The combination diet can substantially reduce blood pressure, and, accordingly, provides an additional lifestyle approach to preventing and treating hypertension."

Adding Dairy Is Easier Than Restricting Salt

As the DASH researchers said, a diet rich in fruits, vegetables, and low-fat dairy products is an additional lifestyle approach, not the only one. High blood pressure has many possible causes and many possible solutions. If you're already consuming 3 servings of dairy a day and you still have high blood pressure, adding even more dairy isn't going to solve your problem. But if you're like most North Americans, you aren't consuming 3 servings of dairy a day, so it's likely that the Calcium Key Weight-Loss Plan will be a good first step in dealing with your high blood pressure. After all, adding foods to your diet is a lot easier than restricting foods like salt, which can boost blood pressure in some people. In fact, the two groups of people most likely to benefit from the pressure-reducing power of the Calcium Key Weight-Loss Plan are those who are salt sensitive: African-Americans and people over 65.

For these groups, salt increases the loss of calcium through the urine, which increases calcitriol. More calcium is pushed into smooth muscle cells, which tighten, raising blood pressure. The calcium-rich plan can help reverse that effect.

Preventing Stroke

High blood pressure is the single most important risk factor for stroke—a lightning bolt to the brain that disables or kills 700,000 Americans every year. The relationship between high blood pressure and stroke is simple and stark: the higher your blood pressure, the higher your risk of stroke. So, if dairy foods can lower blood pressure, they should also lower your risk of stroke. Studies show that's exactly what they do.

In a study published in the journal *Stroke*—the leading scientific journal about this disease—researchers at the Honolulu Heart Program looked at more than 3000 men of Japanese ancestry ages 55 to 88, analyzing their dietary habits over 22 years. They found that men who didn't drink milk had twice the rate of stroke compared to men who drank two or more 8-ounce glasses a day. And the scientists made another observation similar to one you have read about again and again in this book: calcium intake from nondairy sources didn't protect the men from stroke. So, it wasn't just the calcium in milk that was the antistroke factor. It was dairy itself, containing a host of known and unknown nutritional factors, that made the difference.

In another study published in *Stroke,* researchers from Harvard Medical School analyzed the patterns of dietary intake and stroke in more than 85,000 women ages 34 to 59. They found that those with the largest intake of calcium had a 31% lower risk of stroke than those with the smallest intake. Once again, it wasn't just the calcium providing the protection. The "association [of low risk of stroke] with calcium intake was stronger for dairy than for nondairy calcium intake," say the authors.

How does dairy protect against stroke? Linda K. Massey, Ph.D., professor in the Department of Food Science and Human Nutrition at Washington State University, considers this question in an article in the *Journal of Nutrition* that reviews studies on dairy intake and stroke. Massey says dairy lowers blood pressure, but that fact alone can't explain the potency of dairy's stroke-preventing power.

She points out that dairy also reduces *platelet aggregation*. Platelets are microscopic plate-shaped parts of blood cells. Their specialty: they stick together, or aggregate. On the positive side, platelets help blood clot when you have a wound. On the negative side, platelets can form a blood clot in an artery, and an artery-blocking clot is the cause of 80% of all strokes.

Dairy foods also increase levels of *tissue-type plasminogen activator,* or *t-PA,* a chemical that dissolves blood clots. In a study published in *Thrombosis Research,* scientists in France found that among 594 men and women ages 30 to 64, those with the highest consumption of milk also had the highest levels of t-PA, 19% higher in men and 13% higher in women. Women who ate the most cheese had a t-PA level that was 21% higher than women who ate the least, and male cheese-lovers had a t-PA level 8% higher than men who did not eat cheese.

Dairy also reduces insulin resistance. Insulin is a hormone that ushers glucose, or blood sugar (the body's primary energy source) into the cells. When the cells resist insulin, there is more circulating blood sugar and more circulating insulin, as the pancreas pumps out more of the hormone to deal with excess blood sugar. Those higher levels of glucose and insulin in the bloodstream can lead to arterial damage, increasing the risk of stroke.

Dairy foods deliver high levels of the mineral potassium, which can reduce the formation of *free radicals,* destructive molecules that can harm the cells of the arteries.

Dairy is also high in magnesium, a mineral that can keep the muscle cells of the arteries toned, much as you tone the big muscles of your body with exercise.

Metabolic Syndrome: Does Dairy Make the Difference?

In the 1980s, scientists began to notice that millions of Americans had a pattern of health problems that put them at increased risk for heart disease and type II (adult-onset) diabetes. These folks were overweight, had high blood pressure, had high levels of triglycerides, had low levels of the good cholesterol, HDL, and had insulin resistance.

Scientists theorized that since these problems were usually found together, they might not be different diseases. Instead, they might be different expressions of the same disease: a disorder in the body's ability to metabolize—to make appropriate and healthy use of—blood sugar and insulin. They called the problem by various names, including syndrome X, insulin resistance syndrome, and metabolic syndrome. I use metabolic syndrome, because I think it's the most accurate description of the condition.

Since it was first recognized in the 1980s, metabolic syndrome has become increasingly common. As of today, 24% of American adults have it! And it is probably the reason that after decades of decline, the rate of heart disease is once again on the rise.

There are some obvious causes of metabolic syndrome, like smoking and lack of exercise. But the dietary cause of the problem isn't well understood. We do know that dairy foods can control overweight and high blood pressure, two features of metabolic syndrome. Could a diet low in dairy foods be one cause of the problem? That's what a group of scientists conducting the CARDIA Study—Coronary Artery Risk Development in Young Adults—decided to find out.

The researchers were from Harvard Medical School, the University of Minnesota, the University of Oslo in Norway, and many other institutions. From 1985 to 1996 they studied the dietary habits of 3000 people ages 18 to 30. When they analyzed the data, they found that overweight people who consumed the most dairy—35 or more servings a week—were 71% less likely to develop metabolic syndrome than were people who consumed 10 or less servings of dairy a week.

Their study, published in the *Journal of the American Medical Association,* also provided more support for my finding on dairy and overweight. They found that every time dairy products are eaten, the odds of being overweight go down—a 20% lower risk for each daily intake of a dairy food like milk, yogurt, or cheese. If you eat 3 servings of dairy a day, your risk of being overweight decreases by 60%.

It's important to point out that this scientific research does not prove that dairy can prevent metabolic syndrome. The CARDIA study researchers conducted an *epidemiological* study—a study that looks at a large group of people and notices a statistical association between one factor and another, in this case, between high dairy intake and low risk of the metabolic syndrome in people who were overweight. But it will take one or more clinical studies—feeding dairy to one group of people with metabolic syndrome; feeding a nondairy control diet to another group; and seeing if dairy clears up the various factors of the problem, as compared to the control diet—to prove that dairy can reverse the condition. Until those clinical studies are conducted, we can't say with certainty how effective the Calcium Key Weight-Loss Plan will be in reducing your risk of metabolic syndrome. But scientists already know that the single best action you can take is to lose weight. And that's exactly what the CKES will help you do.

Calcium and Colon Cancer: Proof of Protection

Colon cancer—cancer of the lining of the large bowel, or colon—is the #2 cause of cancer deaths in the United States, striking 148,300 people a year and killing 56,600. Can calcium and low-fat dairy foods help prevent the problem? Overwhelmingly, the scientific evidence says yes.

In a study published in *Nutrition and Cancer,* scientists from the Karolinska Institute in Sweden looked at the dietary habits of 61,463 women over 11 years. They found that women with the highest intake of calcium—914 mg a day—had a 28% lower risk of developing colon cancer than women with the lowest intake—486 mg a day. "High calcium intake may lower colorectal cancer risk," they concluded. (Colon cancer is sometimes referred to as colorectal cancer, to indicate it can involve both the colon and the rectum.)

In a study published in the *Journal of the National Cancer Institute,* researchers from Harvard looked at a decade or more of dietary data from 88,000 women and 47,000 men. They found that women who got more than 1250 mg of calcium a day had a 27% lower risk of colon cancer than women who got less than 500 mg; men who got 1250 mg reduced their risk by 42%, compared to men who got 500 mg.

In a study published in the *European Journal of Clinical Nutrition,* researchers from Finland looked at the diets of 10,000 men and women over 24 years. Those who had the highest consumption of milk had a 54% lower risk of developing colon cancer than those with the lowest consumption. In this case, researchers found that nondairy calcium was not protective— another instance where dairy foods are making the difference, not any particular nutrient in dairy.

A study published in *Cancer Causes and Control* found similar results. Researchers at the Fred Hutchinson Cancer Research Center looked at 1993 people with colon cancer and 2410 people without colon cancer. They found that those who consumed the most low-fat dairy foods had 7 to 8 times less risk of colon cancer than those who consumed the least. They also found that those who consumed the most dietary calcium overall (from dairy and other sources) had 6 times less risk of colon cancer than those who consumed the least.

How do dairy and calcium work to prevent colon cancer? Like every cancer, colon cancer begins as normal cells start to divide and multiply abnormally, or *proliferate.* In colon cancer, the cells that proliferate are the *epithelial* cells that line the large intestine. These proliferating cells change in many ways before they turn into cancer. There are more of them, of course; they secrete a different type of mucous; the typical size of the nucleus, or center, of the cells changes; and cellular proteins called *cytokeratins* grow abnormally.

In an article published in the *Journal of the American Medical Association,* researchers at Columbia University looked at whether low-fat dairy products could reverse these early signs of colon cancer in people at high risk for the disease—people with a history of growths in the colon called *polyps.*

They studied 70 people with polyps, dividing them into two main groups: those eating low-fat dairy products containing up to 1200 mg of daily calcium and those not eating dairy. At 6 and 12 months into the study, the researchers measured five indicators of proliferative activity: (1) the number of proliferative cells; (2) the total area of proliferation; (3) the acidity of the mucous membranes; (4) the size of the cell nuclei; and (5) the level of cytokeratins.

Among the group of people eating low-fat dairy foods, every one of those measurements moved "toward that of normal cells," say the researchers. But in those not eating dairy, there was no difference from the level of abnormal cellular activity when the study started. The authors concluded that "Increasing the daily intake of calcium by up to 1200 mg via low-fat dairy food" can stop proliferative changes in the colon and restore all the indicators of normal cell differentiation.

Researchers at Columbia University conducted another similar study. They gave a 900 mg supplement of calcium carbonate or low-fat dairy food with the same amount of calcium to 40 people at high risk for colon cancer. Both the calcium supplements and the dairy decreased a standard measurement (or index) of cell proliferation by about 25% in one part of the colon and by about two-thirds in another section of the large bowel. Writing in *Nutrition and Cancer,* the researchers proclaim the power of dairy and calcium to reverse the early signs of colon cancer.

Breast Cancer and Low-Fat Dairy Foods

There is very preliminary epidemiological evidence that dairy foods and calcium may reduce the risk of breast cancer. Intriguing studies but no definitive proof. What we can say with confidence, however, is that dairy products do not cause breast cancer—something they've been accused of in the low-fat mania that's seized the country for so many years. Here's the research.

In a study in the *Journal of the National Cancer Institute,* researchers at Harvard School of Public Health looked at the dietary history of 88,000 women for 16 years. Among premenopausal women, they found that those who ate the most low-fat dairy foods had a 32% lower risk of developing breast cancer than those who ate the least. And those who drank the most skim or low-fat milk had a 28% lower risk of breast cancer than those who drank the least.

A similar study, conducted by Finnish researchers and published in the *British Journal of Cancer,* looked at the dietary habits of 4697 women over

25 years. Those who drank the most milk had a 58% lower risk of cancer than those who drank the least.

If dairy does protect against breast cancer, what might the mechanism be? Many studies in the laboratory show that vitamin D, an ingredient of milk, can kill breast cancer cells. But much more research is needed before scientists can say whether dairy or any of its components can prevent the disease.

One Study about Ovarian Cancer

A study published in the *American Journal of Epidemiology* showed that consumption of low-fat dairy foods may help prevent ovarian cancer, which kills about 14,000 women a year. This research is even more preliminary than that for breast cancer, but it's certainly worth mentioning in a chapter about dairy foods and health.

The researchers, from the Cancer Research Center of Hawaii at the University of Hawaii, looked at the dietary habits of 558 women with ovarian cancer and 607 women without the disease. They found that those who ate the most dairy products and drank the most milk had the lowest risk of ovarian cancer. They also found that women who had the most calcium in their diets were 64 percent less likely to get ovarian cancer than women who had the least. "These results," say the authors, "suggest that intake [of low-fat milk and calcium] may reduce the risk of ovarian cancer.

Prostate Cancer: Does Dairy Put Men at Risk?

Perhaps you've read in the news that dairy products may actually increase the risk of prostate cancer. I don't share this view, for a number of reasons.

First, the issue was summarized in a comprehensive review of 100 scientific studies on dairy intake and prostate cancer by the American Institute of Cancer Research, a nonprofit organization funding research on diet, nutrition, and cancer. "From a purely scientific standpoint, it would be irresponsible to assert that drinking milk increases a person's risk for prostate cancer in particular," says Helen A. Norman, Ph.D., co-author of the review. The review points out that there is no clear biochemical pathway that could explain how consumption of dairy foods might actually influence the growth of prostate cancer cells.

Second, the only studies indicating risk are epidemiological. (And many other epidemiological studies show no risk.) Epidemiological studies look at a group of people, show a statistical association between two factors in that group, and propose that one factor may have caused the other. But these studies do not provide proof of that cause. All they provide is an intriguing clue for other investigators to follow with studies on cells, tissues, animals, and eventually humans.

Third, evidence shows that rates of prostate cancer among African-Americans—a group at high risk for the disease—are lower among men with the highest consumption of dairy and calcium.

If you're an overweight man thinking about following the Calcium Key Weight-Loss Plan, do not let scare stories about dairy intake and prostate cancer discourage you. There is no scientifically proven threat.

PMS and Calcium

PMS, or premenstrual syndrome, is the #1 reason premenopausal women see their doctors. And no wonder. The common symptoms of PMS include fluid retention, bloating, food cravings, weight gain, skin problems, breast tenderness, mood swings, irritability, anxiety, depression, difficulty concentrating, tearfulness, fatigue, headache, cramps, aching joints, nausea, upset stomach, and insomnia. What could cause all that suffering before a woman's period?

It might be a deficiency of calcium. That's the opinion of Susan Thys-Jacobs, M.D., assistant professor of medicine at Columbia University. This opinion is supported by many scientific studies. In her article "Micronutrients and the Premenstrual Syndrome: The Case for Calcium" published in the *Journal of the American College of Nutrition*, Thys-Jacobs discusses why PMS may be caused by a "calcium deficiency state" and why calcium may be the best treatment for the problem.

The hormone estrogen regulates calcium metabolism, she explains, affecting its absorption and triggering low blood levels of calcium during the menstrual cycle. Studies show that having too little (or much too much) calcium in the blood can cause changes in emotion, like depression, anxiety, and mood swings—the same changes that characterize PMS. In fact, says Thys-Jacobs, the similarity in symptoms between PMS and hypocalcemia—too little calcium—is remarkable. Her conclusion is that the symptoms of PMS are caused by a calcium deficiency that is unmasked when hormones rise during the menstrual cycle.

The theory is backed up by three clinical studies in which calcium tamed the symptoms of PMS. In one study, 33 women with PMS received 3 months of treatment with 1000 mg of calcium, followed by 3 months on a placebo. Seventy-three percent of the women said their symptoms improved while on calcium; statistically, there was an overall 50% reduction in symptoms.

In another study, 10 women with PMS took either 587 mg or 1336 mg of calcium a day. While on the high-calcium intake, the women had improvements in mood, behavior, pain, and water retention.

In the most recent study, conducted at clinics across the United States, 472 women with PMS took either 1200 mg of calcium a day or a placebo for 3 months. Calcium reduced overall symptoms by 48%. It was effective on all four of the core symptom factors of PMS: negative emotions, water retention, food cravings, and pain. And it reduced 15 of the 17 PMS symptoms tracked during the study.

If you have PMS, you probably want to talk to your doctor about increasing your calcium intake. If you're overweight, have PMS, and are trying out the Calcium Key Weight-Loss Plan, you may find your symptoms disappearing along with your pounds.

Hope for Polycystic Ovarian Syndrome

Polycystic ovarian syndrome is one of the leading causes of infertility; 6 to 10% of all women have it, though many don't know it. Its symptoms are similar to metabolic syndrome, but worse: high blood pressure, high insulin levels, overweight, acne, excess hair on the face and body but thinning hair on the scalp, infertility, and usually numerous cysts on the ovaries—cysts that have developed from *follicles*, or maturing eggs.

No one knows what causes PCOS. Thys-Jacobs thinks low levels of calcium could be an important factor. Writing in *Steroids*, she points out that numerous studies show calcium has a key role in the development of the ovaries in the fetus as well as the development of follicles during the menstrual cycle. She questioned if calcium dysregulation could contribute to the arrested follicular development of PCOS.

To test this hypothesis, she gave calcium and vitamin D to 13 women with PCOS. In 2 months, 7 of the women had normal menstrual cycles and 2 became pregnant. That's a remarkable result for this hard-to-treat disease. She concluded, "Abnormalities in calcium . . . may be responsible, in part, for the arrested follicular development in women with PCOS and may contribute to the pathogenesis [development] of PCOS." Not proof by any means but an intriguing hypothesis and study. And perhaps some additional hope for the millions of women with PCOS.

Postpartum Depression: Can Calcium Help?

A study from Oregon Health and Science University provides an intriguing lead for scientists to follow. Postpartum depression (PPD) afflicts 12 to 16% of new mothers, usually a few weeks or months after giving birth. They feel sad nearly all the time. The sadness may last for weeks or months, and these mothers are unable to derive pleasure from things that would ordinarily make them happy, like the baby.

Getting enough sleep, getting breaks from caring for the baby, and remembering to eat regular meals can all help PPD. So can antidepressant medications and cognitive therapy, which helps a new mother understand the thinking and beliefs that underlie her depression. Calcium might help, too.

In a study on preeclampsia—high blood pressure during pregnancy—researchers at Oregon Health and Science University gave women either calcium supplements or a placebo. After the women gave birth, the researchers noticed that fewer of the mothers who took calcium got postpartum depression, as compared to the mothers who took the placebo. They're currently conducting a study focusing on calcium and PPD.

Again, this is not proof. But definitely another reason for pregnant women to make sure they get enough calcium in their diets along with the full array of other nutrients so critical during this time.

Calcium and Kidney Stones

If you have kidney stones, your doctor has probably told you to stay away from high-calcium foods like dairy products. Well, after you read the following section, you might want to have another conversation with your doc about the wisdom of his or her advice. That's because the traditional low-calcium diet to prevent kidney stones is a bad idea. Yes, 80% of kidney stones contain calcium oxalate. And on that basis, most urologists have recommended a low-calcium diet to those who've had a calcium oxalate stone, theorizing it will help prevent a recurrence. That's the wrong approach. Research shows that normal levels of calcium in the diet decrease the level of oxalate in the urine, reducing the risk of oxalate-containing stones.

In research published in the *New England Journal of Medicine*, Italian scientists studied 60 kidney stone formers for 5 years, giving 30 a traditional low-calcium diet and the other 30 a normal level of calcium. At the end of the study, 23 people on the low-calcium diet had formed another kidney stone, compared to 12 getting normal levels.

One caution about calcium does apply, however, for those with kidney stones: don't take calcium supplements, particularly first thing in the morning or at bedtime. This large load of calcium can crystallize fairly easily, perhaps increasing the risk of kidney stones.

Calcium in food can prevent kidney stones, but calcium supplements can cause them. Calcium in low-fat dairy doubles your rate of weight loss; calcium in supplements doesn't. Calcium in dairy is twice as powerful as supplements in lowering high blood pressure. Dairy is just as good as calcium supplements at reversing the precancerous changes of colon cancer—and, say some epidemiological studies, it may be better at preventing the disease. And it is dairy that studies show is best at preventing stroke.

The bottom line of this chapter isn't to say that you gain better health by popping a calcium pill. It's to follow the Calcium Key Weight-Loss Plan and reap all the possible health benefits from that plan: a thinner body, stronger bones, protection against stroke and maybe heart disease, a shield against colon cancer. It's doubly satisfying to know that as you decrease your weight, you're also decreasing your risk for serious illnesses. What could be better?

8

The Calcium Key for Life

HOW OFTEN HAVE you bought a new diet book, put yourself on its strange eating plan, lost weight (exciting!), then dismally watched yourself gain the weight back, pound by pound, because there was no way you could sustain the unusual eating style the diet required? If you're anything like most of us, you've done that over and over and (sigh) over again. Studies show that 85% of people who go on a diet gain back the pounds they lost.

The Calcium Key puts those failures behind you. Now and in the future, you will experience weight-loss success, because you've discovered the missing link in weight loss. You've discovered that simply by adding 3 to 4 servings of calcium-rich dairy to your daily diet, you've changed the way your fat cells function.

Your fat cells now *make less fat.*

Your fat cells now *burn more fat.*

Your fat cells now *store less fat.*

You've learned to use the latest scientific discovery in weight loss—the discovery that explains why so many people have had such a hard time shedding pounds—and put it to work in your own life. You've combined those 3 servings of dairy with just a bit of daily calorie cutting and a bit of exercise, and you've seen the pounds peel away week after week.

The Calcium Key Weight-Loss Plan is very similar in nutritional composition to the diet you were probably already eating, so you can stay on it for the rest of your life. Yes, you can and will keep your excess weight off for the rest of your life!

Not only that, you're now a whole lot healthier. By eating a calcium-rich diet, you're less likely to suffer from heart disease, stroke, diabetes, colon cancer, and osteoporosis.

Congratulations. You've made the smart choice, the scientifically informed choice. The choice to forget about fads and avail yourself of the newest, most significant discovery in practical weight loss.

As you admire your new body in the mirror . . . as you feel better and worry less about chronic disease . . . as the frustrating cycle of weight loss and weight gain becomes a dim memory . . . you'll look back on the day you first used the Calcium Key Weight-Loss Plan to unlock your fat cells—you'll know you also unlocked your natural potential for a lifetime of satisfying slimness and health!

Recommended Reading

Fat Land: How Americans Became the Fattest People in the World. Greg Critser (Houghton-Mifflin, 2003).

An exacting and entertaining description of the obesity epidemic and how it happened.

The New Glucose Revolution: The Authoritative Guide to the Glycemic Index—the Dietary Solution for Lifelong Health. Jeannie Brand-Miller, Thomas M. S. Wolever, Kaye Foster-Powell, and Stephen Colagiuri (Marlow & Company, 2003).

The most authoritative, science-based guide to the glycemic index.

The Volumetrics Weight-Control Plan: Feel Full on Fewer Calories. Barbara Rolls and Robert A. Barnett (Harper Mass Market Paperbacks, 2002).

Smart advice from the leading scientific expert on low-calorie, high-volume eating.

The Official Pocket Guide to Diabetic Exchanges. American Diabetes Association. American Dietetic Association (McGraw-Hill/Contemporary Distributed Products, 1998).

Although diabetic exchanges are not the same as the Calcium Key Exchange System, this book can be useful in helping you determine your daily exchanges.

ACSM Fitness Book, 3rd edition. American College of Sports Medicine (Human Kinetics, 2003).

"A common-sense, science-based, step-by-step approach to becoming active and fit," says Dixie Thompson, the fitness consultant for The Calcium Key.

Notes

Introduction

Calle EE, et al. "Overweight, obesity, and mortality from cancer in a prospectively studied cohort of U.S. adults." *New England Journal of Medicine.* 2003;348(17):1625–1638.

"Clinical Guidelines on the Identification, Evaluation, and Treatment of Overweight and Obesity in Adults." National Heart, Lung and Blood Institute.

Critser, Greg. *Fat Land: How Americans Became the Fattest People in the World.* Houghton Mifflin, 2003.

Heaney RP. "Normalizing calcium intake: projected population effects for body weight." *Journal of Nutrition.* 2003;133(1):268S–270S.

Kurth T, et al. Body mass index and the risk of stroke in men. *Archives of Internal Medicine.* 2002;162(22):2557–2562.

Nielsen SJ, et al. "Patterns and trends in food portion sizes, 1977–1998." *Journal of the American Medical Association.* 2003;289:450–453.

"Obesity Epidemic Increases Dramatically in the United States." National Center for Chronic Disease Prevention and Health. Centers for Disease Control and Prevention. http://www.cdc.gov/nccdphp/dnpa/obesity-epidemic.htm.

Ogden CL, et al. "Prevalence and Trends in Overweight Among US Children and Adolescents, 1999–2000." *Journal of the American Medical Association.* 2002;288:14,1728–32.

"Overweight and Obesity: Health Consequences." Centers for Disease Control and Prevention. http://www.cdc.gov/nccdphp/dnpa/obesity/consequences.htm.

"Overweight and Obesity: The Surgeon General's Call to Action to Prevent and Decrease Overweight and Obesity." http://www.surgeongeneral.gov/topics/obesity/calltoaction/fact_consequences.htm.

"Physical Activity Among Adults: United States, 2000." National Center for Health Statistics, Centers for Disease Control and Prevention, U.S. Department of Health and Human Services.

U.S. Obesity Trends: 1985 to 2001. National Center for Chronic Disease Prevention and Health. Centers for Disease Control and Prevention. http://www.cdc.gov/nccdphp/dnpa/obesity/trend/maps/.

"What We Eat in America." United States Department of Agriculture.

Zemel MB. Role of dietary calcium and dairy products in modulating adiposity. *Lipids.* 2003;38(2):139–146.

Chapter 1. Discovering the Calcium–Fat Connection

Davies KM, et al. "Calcium intake and body weight." *Journal of Clinical Endocrinology and Metabolism.* 2000;85:4635–4638.

Lin Y-C, et al. "Dairy calcium is related to changes in body composition during a two-year exercise intervention in young women. *Journal of the American College of Nutrition.* 2000;19(6):715.

McCarron DA, et al. "Dietary calcium in human hypertension." *Science.* 1982;217(4556):267–269.

McCarron DA, et al. "Blood pressure and nutrient intake in the United States." *Science.* 1984;224(4656):1392–1398.

Shi H, et al. "Role of the sulfonylurea receptor in regulating human adipocyte metabolism." *FASEB Journal.* 1999;13(13):1833–1838.

Shi H, et al. "Role of intracellular calcium in human adipocyte differentiation." *Physiological Genomics.* 2000;3(2):75–82.

Shi H, et al. "Effects of dietary calcium on adipocyte lipid metabolism and body weight regulation in energy-restricted aP2-agouti transgenic mice." *FASEB Journal.* 2001;15(2):291–293.

Sun X, et al. "Calcium and dairy inhibition of weight and fat regain during ad libitum feeding following energy restriction in aP2-agouti transgenic mice." *FASEB Journal.* 2003;17A746

Xue B, Zemel MB. "Relationship between human adipose tissue agouti and fatty acid synthase (FAS)." *American Society for Nutritional Sciences.* 2000;22:3166.

Xue B, et al. "The *agouti* gene product inhibits lipolysis in human adipocytes via a Ca2+-dependent mechanism." *FASEB Journal.* 1998;12(13): 1391–1396.

Zemel MB. "Mechanisms of dairy modulation of adiposity." *Journal of Nutrition.* 2003;133(1):252S–256S.

Zemel MB, et al. "Regulation of adiposity by dietary calcium." *FASEB Journal.* 2000;14(9):1132–1138.

Zemel MB, et al. "Dietary calcium and dairy products accelerate weight and fat loss during energy restriction in obese adults." *American Journal of Clinical Nutrition.* 2002;75(suppl):342S.

Chapter 2. Unlocking Your Fat Cells

Anderson JW, et al. "Health advantages and disadvantages of weight-reducing diets: computer analysis and critical reviews." *Journal of the American College of Nutrition.* 2000;19(5):578–590.

Boutelle KN, et al. "Further support for consistent self-monitoring as a vital component of successful weight control." *Obesity Research.* 1998;6(3): 219–224.

Brand-Miller J, Wolever TMS, Foster-Powell K, Colagiuri S. *The New Glucose Revolution.* Marlowe & Company (2003).

Bravata DM, et al. Efficacy and safety of low-carbohydrate diets: a systematic review. *Journal of the American Medical Association.* 2003;289(14): 1837–1850.

Case CC, et al. "Impact of weight loss on the metabolic syndrome." *Diabetes and Obesity Metabolism.* 2002;4(6):407–414.

Hankey CR, et al. "Effects of moderate weight loss on anginal symptoms and indices of coagulation and fibrinolysis in overweight patients with angina pectoris." *European Journal of Clinical Nutrition.* 2002;56(10): 1039–1045.

Himaya A, et al. "The effect of soup on satiation." *Appetite.* 1998;30(2): 199–210.

Jenkins DJ, et al. "Glycemic index of foods: a physiological basis for carbohydrate exchange. *American Journal of Clinical Nutrition.* 1981;34: 362–366.

Jenkins D, et al. "Glycemic index: overview of implications in health and disease." *American Journal of Clinical Nutrition.* July 2002;76(1): 266S–273S.

Landers P, et al. "Effect of weight loss plans on body composition and diet duration." *Journal of the Oklahoma State Medical Association.* 2002; 95(5):329–331.

Latner JD, et al. "Effective long-term treatment of obesity: a continuing care model." *International Journal of Obesity and Related Metabolic Disorders.* 2000;24(7):893–898.

Ludwig DS. "The glycemic index: physiological mechanisms relating to obesity, diabetes, and cardiovascular disease." *Journal of the American Medical Association.* 2002;287:2414–2423.

Ludwig DS, et al. "Dietary fiber, weight gain, and cardiovascular disease risk factors in young adults." *Journal of the American Medical Association.* 1999;282(16):1539–1546.

Morris, KL, Zemel MB. "Glycemic index, cardiovascular disease, and obesity." *Nutrition Reviews.* 1999;57(9 Pt 1):273–276.

Rolls BJ, et al. "Water incorporated into a food but not served with a food decreases energy intake in lean women." *American Journal of Clinical Nutrition.* 1999;70(4):448–455.

Sartorio A, et al. "Short-term changes of cardiovascular risk factors after a non-pharmacological body weight reduction program." *European Journal of Clinical Nutrition.* 2001;55(10):865–869.

Taubes, G. "The soft science of dietary fat." *Science.* 2001;291(5513): 2536–2545.

"Volumetrics: Feel Full on Fewer Calories." Barbara Rolls, Ph.D., and Robert A. Barnett (HarperCollins, 2000).

Willett WC, et al. "Dietary fat is not a major determinant of body fat." *American Journal of Medicine.* 2002;113(Suppl 9B):47S–59S.

Yoshioka M, et al. "Combined effects of red pepper and caffeine consumption on 24 h energy balance in subjects given free access to foods." *British Journal of Nutrition.* 2001;85(2):203–211.

Chapter 3. Calcium Key Weight-Loss Success

Barillas C, et al. Effective reduction of lactose maldigestion in preschool children by direct addition of beta-galactosidases to milk at mealtime. *Pediatrics* 1987;79(5):766–772.

Dehkordi N, et al. "Lactose malabsorption as influenced by chocolate milk, skim milk, sucrose, whole milk, and lactic cultures." *Journal of the American Dietetic Association.* 1995;95(4):484–486.

Hertzler SR, et al. "Colonic adaptation to daily lactose feeding in lactose maldigesters reduces lactose intolerance." *American Journal of Clinical Nutrition.* 1996;64(2):232–236.

Hertzler SR, et al. "How much lactose is low lactose?" *Journal of the American Dietetic Association.* 1996;96(3):243–246.

Jiang T, et al. "In vitro lactose fermentation by human colonic bacteria is modified by *Lactobacillus acidophilus* supplementation." *Journal of Nutrition.* 1997;127(8):1489–1495.

Kolars JC, et al. "Yogurt—an autodigesting source of lactose." *New England Journal of Medicine.* 1984;310(1):1–3.

Lami F, et al. "Efficacy of addition of exogenous lactase to milk in adult lactase deficiency." *American Journal of Gastroenterology.* 1988;83(10): 1145–1149.

Lee CM, et al. Cocoa feeding and human lactose intolerance. *American Journal of Clinical Nutrition.* 1989;49(5):840–844.

Lin MY, et al. "Comparative effects of exogenous lactase (beta-galactosidase) preparations on in vivo lactose digestion." *Digestive Diseases and Sciences.* 1993;38(11):2022–2027.

Martini MC, et al. "Reduced intolerance symptoms from lactose consumed during a meal." *American Journal of Clinical Nutrition.* 1988;47(1):57–60.

Mustapha A, et al. "Improvement of lactose digestion by humans following ingestion of unfermented acidophilus milk: influence of bile sensitivity, lactose transport, and acid tolerance of *Lactobacillus acidophilus.*" *Journal of Dairy Science.* 1997;80(8):1537–1545.

Pribila BA, et al. "Improved lactose digestion and intolerance among African-American adolescent girls fed a dairy-rich diet." *Journal of the American Dietetic Association.* 2000;100(5):524–528.

Rosado JL, et al. "Enzyme replacement therapy for primary adult lactase deficiency. Effective reduction of lactose malabsorption and milk intolerance by direct addition of beta-galactosidase to milk at mealtime." *Gastroenterology.* 1984;87(5):1072–1082.

Shermak MA, et al. "Effect of yogurt on symptoms and kinetics of hydrogen production in lactose-malabsorbing children." *American Journal of Clinical Nutrition.* 1995;62(5):1003–1006.

Suarez FL, et al. "A comparison of symptoms after the consumption of milk or lactose-hydrolyzed milk by people with self-reported severe lactose intolerance." *New England Journal of Medicine.* 1995;333(1):1–4.

Suarez FL, et al. "Tolerance to the daily ingestion of two cups of milk by individuals claiming lactose intolerance." *American Journal of Clinical Nutrition.* 1997;65(5):1502–1506.

Suarez FL, et al. "Lactose maldigestion is not an impediment to the intake of 1500 mg calcium daily as dairy products." *American Journal of Clinical Nutrition.* 1998;68:1118–1122.

Vesa TH, et al. "Tolerance to small amounts of lactose in lactose maldigesters." *American Journal of Clinical Nutrition.* 1996;64(2): 197–201.

Vesa TH, et al. "Lactose intolerance." *Journal of the American College of Nutrition.* 2000;19(900002):165S–175S.

Chapter 6. Burn More Fat with Easy Exercise

Andersen RE, et al. Effects of lifestyle activity vs structured aerobic exercise in obese women: a randomized trial. *Journal of the American Medical Association.* 1999;281(4):335–340.

Anderson JW, et al. "Long-term weight-loss maintenance: a meta-analysis of US studies." 2001;74(5):579–584.

Asikainen TM, et al. "Walking trials in postmenopausal women: effect of one vs two daily bouts on aerobic fitness." *Scandinavian Journal of Medicine and Science in Sports.* 2002;12(2):99–105.

Irwin ML, et al. "Effect of exercise on total and intra-abdominal body fat in postmenopausal women: a randomized controlled trial." 2003;289(3): 323–330.

Jakicic JM, et al. "Effects of intermittent exercise and use of home exercise equipment on adherence, weight loss, and fitness in overweight women: a randomized trial." *Journal of the American Medical Association.* 1999;282(16):1554–1560.

Jakicic JM, et al. "Appropriate intervention strategies for weight loss and prevention of weight regain for adults." American College of Sports Medicine. Position Stand. *Medicine & Science in Sports & Exercise.* 2001; 0195–9131:3312–2145.

Kiernan M, et al. "Men gain additional psychological benefits by adding exercise to a weight-loss program." *Obesity Research.* 2001;9(12): 770–777.

Moreau KL, et al. "Increasing daily walking lowers blood pressure in post-menopausal women." *Medicine & Science in Sports & Exercise.* 2001;33(11):1825–1831.

Nieman DC, et al. "Psychological response to exercise training and/or energy restriction in obese women." *Journal of Psychosomatic Research.* 2000;48(1):23–29.

Schmidt WD, et al. "Effects of long versus short bout exercise on fitness and weight loss in overweight females." *Journal of the American College of Nutrition.* 2001;20(5):494–501.

Chapter 7. Gaining Health While Losing Weight

Abbott RD, et al. "Effect of dietary calcium and milk consumption on risk of thromboembolic stroke in older middle-aged men. The Honolulu Heart Program." *Stroke.* 1996;27:813–818.

Bierenbaum ML, et al. "The effect of dietary calcium supplementation on blood pressure and serum lipid levels." *Nutrition Reports International.* 1987;36:1147–1157.

Borghi L, et al. Comparison of two diets for the prevention of recurrent stones in idiopathic hypercalciuria. 2002;346(2):77–84.

Bucher HC, et al. "Effects of dietary calcium supplementation on blood pressure. A meta-analysis of randomized controlled trials." *Journal of the American Medical Association.* 1996;275:1016–1022.

Goodman MT, et al. "Association of dairy products, lactose, and calcium with the risk of ovarian cancer." *American Journal of Epidemiology.* 2002;156(2):148–157.

Harsha DW, et al. "Dietary approaches to stop hypertension: a summary of study results. DASH Collaborative Research Group." *Journal of the American Dietetic Association.* 1999;99(8 Suppl):S35–39.

Hatton, D. Associate Professor in Behavioral Neuroscience, Oregon Health & Science University. "The use of calcium supplements during pregnancy to reduce incidence of postpartum depression in new mothers." New clinical trial.

Heaney RP, et al. "Effect of yogurt on a urinary marker of bone resorption in postmenopausal women." *Journal of the American Medical Association.* 2002;102:1672–1673.

Holt PR, et al. "Modulation of abnormal colonic epithelial cell proliferation and differentiation by low-fat dairy foods: a randomized controlled trial." *Journal of the American Medical Association.* 1998;280(12): 1074–1079.

Holt PR, et al. "Comparison of calcium supplementation or low-fat dairy foods on epithelial cell proliferation and differentiation." *Nutrition and Cancer.* 2001;41(1–2):150–155.

Iso H, et al. "Prospective study of calcium, potassium, and magnesium intake and risk of stroke in women." *Stroke*. 1999;30:1772–1779.

Jarvinen R, et al. "Prospective study on milk products, calcium and cancers of the colon and rectum." *European Journal of Clinical Nutrition*. 2001;55(11):1000–1007.

Kalkwarf HJ, et al. "Milk intake during childhood and adolescence, adult bone density, and osteoporotic fractures in US women." *American Journal of Clinical Nutrition*. 2003;77(1):257–265.

Kampman E, et al. "Calcium, vitamin D, sunshine exposure, dairy products and colon cancer risk (United States)." *Cancer Causes and Control*. 2000; 11(5):459–466.

Knekt P, et al. "Intake of dairy products and the risk of breast cancer." *British Journal of Cancer*. 1996;73(5):687–691.

Massey LK. "Dairy food consumption, blood pressure and stroke." *Journal of Nutrition*. 2001;131:1875–1878.

Mennen LI, et al. "Tissue-type plasminogen activator antigen and consumption of dairy products. The D.E.S.I.R. Study." *Thrombosis Research*. 1999;94:381–388.

Norman HA, Butrum R. "Is Milk a Risk Factor for Prostate Cancer? An Assessment of the Literature." American Institute for Cancer Research. February 26, 2002.

"Osteoporosis Prevention, Diagnosis, and Therapy." National Institutes of Health Consensus Development Conference Statement. 2000 March 27–29;17(1):1–36. http://consensus.nih.gov/cons/111/111_statement. htm.

Pereira MA, et al. "Dairy consumption, obesity, and the insulin resistance syndrome in young adults. The CARDIA Study." *Journal of the American Medical Association*. 2002;287(16):2081–2089.

Shea B, et al. "Meta-analyses of therapies for postmenopausal osteoporosis. VII. Meta-analysis of calcium supplementation for the prevention of postmenopausal osteoporosis." *Endocrine Reviews*. 2002;23(4):552–559.

Shin MH, et al. "Intake of dairy products, calcium, and vitamin D and risk of breast cancer." *Journal of the National Cancer Institute*. 2002; 94(17):1301–1311.

Terry P, et al. "Dietary calcium and vitamin D intake and risk of colorectal cancer: a prospective cohort study in women." *Nutrition and Cancer*. 2002;43(1):39–46.

Thys-Jacob, S, "Micronutrients and the premenstrual syndrome: the case for calcium." *Journal of the American College of Nutrition.* 2000;19(2):220–227.

Thys-Jacob S, et al. "Vitamin D and calcium dysregulation in the polycystic ovarian syndrome." *Steroids.* 1999;64(6):430–435.

Wu K, et al. "Calcium intake and risk of colon cancer in women and men." *Journal of the National Cancer Institute.* 2002;94(6):437–446.

Zemel MB, et al. "Effect of sodium and calcium on calcium metabolism and blood pressure regulation in hypertensive black adults as affected by dietary calcium and sodium." *Journal of Hypertension.* 1986;4(suppl 5):S343–S345.

Zemel MB, et al. "Reductions in total and extracellular water associated with calcium-induced natriuresis and the antihypertensive effect of calcium in blacks." *American Journal of Hypertension.* 1988;1:70–72.

Index